Charles N. Pappas

The Life and Times of G. V. Black

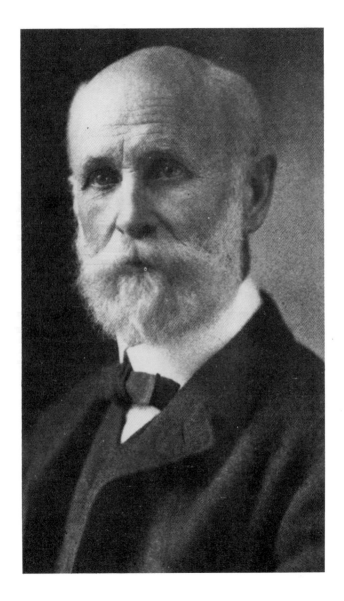

The Life and Times of G.V. Black

Charles N. Pappas, D.D.S.
Assistant Professor of Restorative Dentistry
School of Dental Medicine
University of Pennsylvania, Philadelphia, Pennsylvania

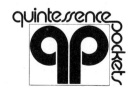
quintessence pockets

Copyright © 1983 Quintessence Publishing Co., Inc., Chicago
Composition: Beslow, Chicago
Printing and Binding: North Central Publ. Co., St. Paul, MN
Printed in U.S.A.
ISBN-0-931386-55-1

Acknowledgments

The author acknowledges with gratitude his indebtedness to the following authors and copyright owners for their kind permission to include quotations from the works designated in the following:

Dr. Carl E. Black, III:
  Carl E. Black's and Bessie M. Black's From Pioneer to Scientist, published by Bruce Publishing Company, 1940.
George Allen and Unwin, Ltd.:
  Contemporary American Philosophy, Second Series, ed. by John E. Smith, 1970.
Harper & Row:
  John E. Smith's Themes in American Philosophy, 1970.
The MacMillan Company:
  F. S. C. Northrop's The Taming of the Nations, published by the Hafner Publishing Company, Inc., 1952.
Muriel Rukeyser's:
  Willard Gibbs, Copyright 1942 © Muriel Rukeyser, Copyright 1970 © Muriel Rukeyser.
I am grateful and indebted as well to the following owners of copyrights for their kind permission to reproduce illustrations as indicated:
Dr. Carl E. Black, III for all of the illustrations which are from Carl E. Black's and Bessie M. Black's From Pioneer to Scientist, with the exception of the illustrations listed.

Mrs. Carl E. Black, II for Figure 28, the illustration of G. V. Black's paper "Civilization."

Mrs. Nora Sigerist Beeson for Figure 18, the four photographs in this figure from Dr. Henry Sigerist's The Great Doctors.

The illustrations in Figure 16 are from the American Textbook of Operative Dentistry, 1897; The Principles and Practice of Dentistry, 12th Ed., 1889; and The Dental Cosmos, Vol XX, 1878.

Thanks are extended to Mr. David J. Sullivan, Photographer of the School of Dental Medicine of the University of Pennsylvania, for his expert photographic reproduction of the illustrations, and to Mr. Bernie Moser, Dufor Photographic Studios, Philadelphia, for the photograph of the writer.

Special thanks are also due to Miss Minnie Orfanos, Librarian of The Dental School of Northwestern University, to Mr. John Whittock, Head Librarian of the School of Dental Medicine of the University of Pennsylvania, and assistant librarians, for their kind help in locating and in making available reference material for this article, to the Charles Patterson Van Pelt Library, the Main Library of the University of Pennsylvania, and to the Drexel University Library for the use of materials from their collections.

Further thanks are given to: Mr. H. W. Haase, publisher, Quintessence Publishing Co., Inc., himself a vigorous pioneer in publishing high quality pocket-sized books and color-illustrated credit course literature for self-continuing dental education; Mr. Henry M. Koehler, editor, for his sustained interest, infinite patience, and hard work in editing this book; Mr. Michael Kraft, production director of Quintessence Publishing Co. and staff for the spirit of "follow-through" manifested in completing a high quality production of this book; and for all who have expressed an interest in this work or who had a part, either directly or indirectly, in making it possible, thanks are given!

Finally, I wish to thank my excellent wife, Edith, née Basedow, for her valued opinions on the text and her patient assistance with the typing of the manuscript.

Table of Contents

Chapter 1

Chicago's Guest of Honor

In the last decade of his life, Dr. Greene Vardiman ("G. V.") Black (frontispiece) was honored at a testimonial banquet which was given by the Chicago Odontographic Society in the Gold Room of the Congress Hotel in Chicago on January 29, 1910. More than four hundred of the most distinguished dentists from all parts of the world were present (Fig. 1).

One of the speakers at that banquet, Dr. R. Ottolengui, an editor and contributor to dental literature, from New York City, made the following presentation:

"The Second District Dental Society of New York, having learned of a banquet to be given to Dr. Greene V. Black of the city of Chicago on the evening of January 29, 1910, we, the undersigned, take advantage of the occasion to present a slight token of our appreciation of his life-time labor in the field of scientific dentistry, as dental investigator, bacteriologist, pathologist, and teacher of dentistry. We admire him especially for his great achievements, First, in solving the problem of the relation of caries to hard and soft teeth; second, in solving the problem of the scientific filling of teeth with amalgam and with gold; third, especially, for the doctrine of "Extension for Prevention" by which he created a system of scientific cavity preparation. For this and other practical benefits resulting from his experiments and studies, the Second District Dental Society is everlastingly indebted to him."*

*Black and Black, p. 315

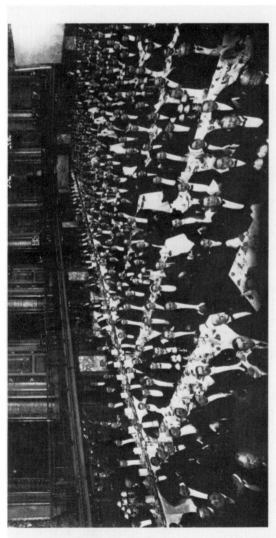

TESTIMONIAL BANQUET GIVEN BY THE CHICAGO ODONTOGRAPHIC SOCIETY IN HONOR OF DR. GREENE V. BLACK, IN THE GOLD ROOM OF THE CONGRESS HOTEL, CHICAGO, ILLINOIS.

Figure 1

This statement was signed by one hundred of Dr. Black's admirers in the East. Dr. Ottolengui continued: "But in addition to this we wanted to bring Dr. Black, our honored guest, some fitting token of our love, of our esteem and of our appreciation, and to me the lot fell of the selection of this gift, and I am glad that our attention was called earlier in the evening to the fact that Mrs. Black is in the audience, because a wise man has said that his pity goes out to the wife of the man of science, because his career will deprive her of much of his society. And when I was thinking of what would be appropriate to bring to Dr. Black I consulted my own wife on the matter. She said, 'I will tell you exactly what to buy for Dr. Black, buy something he would like to look at but something Mrs. Black can make use of.' So, Dr. Black, as your services to the dental profession have been golden, we have thought it proper to present you with a golden coffee service (Fig. 2)."*

The banquet report notes that Dr. Ottolengui's tribute for several reasons brought the greatest round of applause. It was described as:

". . . one of those rare and hearty tributes of the East to the West; a tribute of a great organized city to the earnest student from the country."**

Dr. A. W. Thornton, in attempting to account for G. V. Black's great achievements, included this poem in his remarks:

The heights by great men reached and kept,
Were not attained by sudden flight,
But they while their companions slept,
Were toiling upwards in the night.***

---

*Ibid., p. 316
**Ibid., p. 316
***Anon. (1910), p. 128

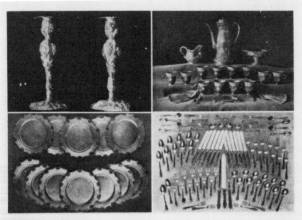

GIFTS PRESENTED TO GREENE V. BLACK.

Silver candlesticks presented by the Dental Faculty, University of Pittsburgh. Gold coffee service presented by second District Dental Society and one hundred professional friends in the East. Silver plates presented by members of the Faculty of Dental Schools, the G. V. Black Club of Saint Paul, the Des Moines and Dubuque Dental Clubs, the Illinois State Board of Dental Examiners and other friends. Chest of Versailles silver presented by the dentists of Illinois.

Figure 2

Dr. Henry W. Morgan of Nashville, Tennessee, gave the South's tribute to G. V. Black and he attempted to describe the great abilities and gifts with which Dr. Black had been endowed with these lines:

"A spirit serene: —
A strength for the daily task.
Courage to face the road;
Good cheer to help the traveler's load.
And for hours to rest that come between,
And inward joy in all things heard and seen."*

*Ibid., p. 134

Finally, after all of the speakers had had their say, the guest of honor was called upon to speak. The report continues:

". . . in a characteristic modest way, (G. V. Black) framed his thanks briefly to the men who had gathered to do him honor. In closing he gave expression to the chief thought that was in his mind when he said that he did not have a goodbye for his friends but rather a good night. He said though he had passed the mark of three score and ten, that he did not believe that his work was over—that there were many things in his mind that ought to be done and that he hoped he might be able to do them. 'I love the work I have been doing and I am not ready to quit.'"

"And so it was given to him even in the years following to accomplish still other great things for the profession to which he had unsacrificingly given the best years of his life."*

The Guest of Honor in Jacksonville, Illinois

At a similar banquet given on April 10, 1911, in his old home town of Jacksonville, Illinois, to which not only members of the dental and medical professions and old friends of thirty-five years, but also the public, were invited, after thanking his audience for the tribute which they had paid him, Dr. G. V. Black said:**

". . . My work has not been all smooth, for much of it has been done over rough ways, and I have often been compelled to retrace my steps. I have made it a habit of my life when I went with a subject as far as I could to drop it and take up some other subject and later go

*Obituary, p. 3
**Black and Black, p. 322

back to the first study. Amid discouragements, I was impelled in some way to go and now at seventy-five, I do not feel that all my work is done although I know the time is short. Things are coming on which will change the whole face of dental treatment, and I believe that succeeding years will bring to pass many changes . . . Anything which perpetuates friendship is valuable. Again, let me thank you."

G. V. Black: what kind of person was he? What had he accomplished that had made him so famous, so respected, and so honored? As we shall see, the answer to each of these questions is perhaps fourfold.

Chapter 2

Nature and Science

Greene Vardiman Black was an energetic, artistic, inventive, creative pioneer who related himself harmoniously to nature—initially through direct experience and observation and later through the study of deductively formulated science.

American Pioneer Saga of the South and North

The progress of the Black family is an American pioneer saga of the South and the North. It is a saga which begins in the South and winds its way through many of the Southern states. It develops further in the North—chiefly in Illinois, and it continues its progress beyond American shores to an international importance in the life of G. V. Black.

G. V. Black's pioneer ancestors arrived in Virginia during colonial times (Fig. 3). There they had to struggle with all of the problems of settling the New World.

Northrop writes: "The key to the people of the United States is that unlike their contemporaries born in older cultures of the world, they were confronted in the Western hemisphere with virgin nature. Thus, nature made by God, rather than the social isms at which traditional cultures have arrived, became their guide and mentor. As Longfellow said, instead of being taught merely by the books of men, they '. . . *read what is still unread in the manuscripts of God.'*

"It is primarily from nature and only secondarily from

The arrival of the settlers at Jamestown in 1607. (A painting by Griffith Baily Coale in the State Capitol, Richmond, Va.)

culture that the spirit of the people of the United States drinks its living waters. In his Phi Beta Kappa address, delivered at Harvard in 1837, Emerson said, 'The first in time and the first in importance in the influences upon the mind is that of nature.'*"

G. V. Black's great-grandfather, William Black, held the rank of captain of the North Carolina Militia shortly before the date of the Mecklenburg Declaration in Charlotte, North Carolina, in the year 1775 (Fig. 4). The Captain was one of the first officers to refuse to take an oath of allegiance to the British Crown.

Captain William Black was also a leader of the Black-Campbell Clan. The forebearers of the Blacks and the Campbells probably migrated directly to North Carolina from Virginia. The Campbells of the Black-Campbell Clan were believed to be members of the same family as the famous Colonel William Campbell, the American Commander of the Mountain Men who had come from North Carolina, South Carolina, and Virginia to fight against Furgeson's British troops on the border between North and South Carolina in the first decisive patriot victory of the American Revolution, Battle of King's Mountain October 7, 1780 (Figs. 5a, b). "Barbarians," Furgeson called these pioneer backwoodsmen and mountaineers as they dealt his forces a crushing defeat. King's Mountain National Military Park, South Carolina, commemorates this famous battle.

*Northrop(a), p. 318

Fig. 3   The Godspeed 40 tons, the Susan Constant 100 tons, and the Discovery 20 tons. G. V. Black's ancestors arrived in Virginia in Colonial times.

19

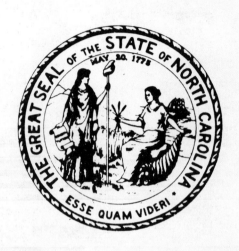

Fig. 4 The figures on the seal represent Liberty (holding a scroll entitled "Constitution") and Plenty. The date on the Great Seal of North Carolina, May 20, 1775, is that of the first Mecklenburg Declaration. G. V. Black's great-grandfather, William Black, was a captain of the North Carolina Militia just before that date (Thorpe).

Fig. 5a Capt. William Black was a leader of the Black-Campbell clan. The Campbells probably were related to Col. (later Gen.) William Campbell, the American commander at the Battle of King's Mountain, fiercely fought, but as time passed, the bond of peace and friendship ultimately prevailed. (This illustration, by F. C. Yohn, was published originally in "The Story of the Revolution" by Henry Cabot Lodge, New York, Charles Scribner's Sons, 1898).

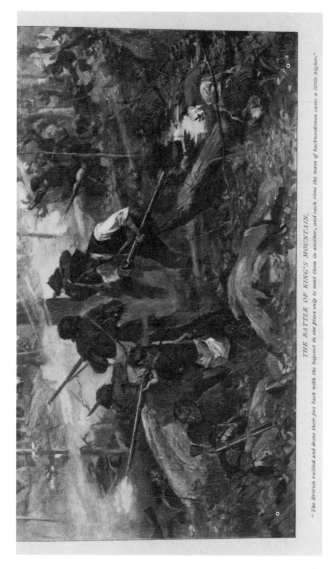

THE BATTLE OF KING'S MOUNTAIN.

"The British rallied and drove their foes back with the bayonet in one place only to meet them in another, and each time the wave of backwoodsmen came a little higher."

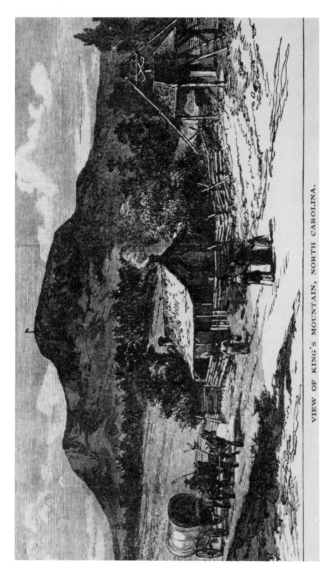

VIEW OF KING'S MOUNTAIN, NORTH CAROLINA.

The courageous, idealistic, ready-to-migrate-to-another-unsettled-country pioneer spirit of these people always saw better opportunities beyond. These mountaineers were prosperous pioneer people. They were not poor.

The frontier people loved to gather to listen to the stories of their great pioneer heroes, such as Colonel William Campbell, Boone, Sevier, and later, General Andrew Jackson. Captain William Black's son, T. G. Black, served as a captain under Andrew Jackson. Doubtless these stories had a powerful effect on their audiences in nourishing the pioneer spirit.

This statement by Raymond Fosdick describes the pioneer way of life:

"The only life worth living at any time in any age is the adventurous life. Now by the adventurous life I mean primarily a life that has a capacity to be different. I mean a life that is willing to cut loose from the past for the sake of the future, that will take chances in casting off from old traditions and old techniques. I mean by the adventurous life a life unwilling to remain tied up in any port, preferring to ride the high seas in search of fairer lands—a life that finds serenity in growth."*

In the same book, Frederick J. Turner, an authority on "The Frontier in American History," adds:

*Black and Black, p. 14

Fig. 5b   During their western migration, members of the Black-Campbell clan told and retold the stories of the pioneer heroes who fought the Battle of King's Mountain. (Illustration from "King's Mountain and its Heroes" by Lyman C. Draper, published by Peter G. Thomson, Cincinnati, 1881).

AN
ACCOUNT
OF TWO
VOYAGES
TO
NEW-ENGLAND.

Wherein you have the setting out of a Ship, With the charges; The prices of all necessaries for furnishing a Planter & his Family at his first coming; A Description of the Country, Natives and Creatures; The Government of the Countrey as it is now possessed by the *English*, &c. A large Chronological Table of the most remarkable passages from the first discovering of the Continent of *America*, to the year 1673.

By *John Josselyn* Gent.

The Second Addition.

Memner. distich rendred English by Dr. *Heylin*.
Heart, take thine ease,
Men hard to please
  Thou haply might'st offend,
Though one speak ill
Of thee, some will
  Say better; there's an end.

London Printed for G. *Widdowes* at the *Green Dragon* in St. *Pauls* Church-yard, 1675.

"All American experience has gone to the making of the spirit of innovation; it is in the blood and will not be repressed."

And also: "In place of old frontiers of wilderness, there are frontiers of unwon fields of science. . ."

With all of the pioneering innovation which was at the core of the spirit of the American frontier, G. V. Black would respond to the challenge of the adventurous life on the "frontier of unwon fields of science" in the field of dentistry.

The American Dental Problem in 1672

Perhaps the earliest statement of the American dental problem was made in 1672 by John Josselyn in his book, *An Account of Two Voyages to New-England, Made during the years 1638, 1663*. In his journal-log (Fig. 6) of these early voyages, Josselyn carefully recorded this observation:

"Men and Women keep their complexions, but lose their Teeth: the Women are pittifully Tooth-shaken; whether through coldness of the climate, or by sweetmeats of which they have store, I am not able to affirm, . . ." (p. 142 of 1865 edition published by William Veazie, Boston).

This recorded early observation was the small, but necessary, important first step toward finding a scientific solution to the dental problem in America. The first

Fig. 6   Title page of Josselyn's book, in which is found the first statement of the American dental problem.

necessary step in initiating any scientific inquiry is making a clear statement of the problem which is to be investigated.

The 'Problem-Tight Compartments of Science'

Sir William Osler, the great physician, teacher of medicine, and author, in his small book, A Way of Life, wrote of the wisdom of "life in 'day-tight' and even 'hour-tight' compartments." By this he seems to have meant: Learn from the past? Yes! Plan for the future? Yes! But dwell negatively on either the past or the future? No! It was a reaffirmation of living the day at hand to its completion.

It was in the act of working quietly, confidently, and steadfastly in the "problem-tight compartments" of dental practice and research that G. V. Black was to be challenged to marshal and to bring to bear nothing less than the full force of all of his powerful interests in observing and studying the natural world about him. In so doing, he would bring into clear focus and complete successfully the purposeful mission of his life and work: the scientific solution to the American dental problem.

G. V. Black's Parents

William Black (born in Milledgeville, Georgia, in 1796), a cabinetmaker by trade, and Mary S. Vaughn, the parents of G. V. Black, met at a singing school in Tennessee and were soon married (Fig. 7). The year was 1825.

The Blacks had been married about nine years when

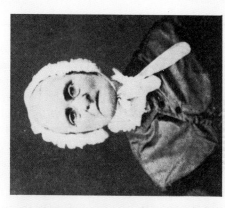

MARY VAUGHN BLACK
1803-1881

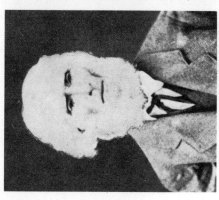

WILLIAM BLACK
1796-1884

Figure 7

27

the Black-Campbell Clan migrated by boat to Naples, Illinois, and landed there on April 13, 1834.*

William and Mary Black left the Tennessee clan and settled thirty miles away from the nearest member. Thus, for the Blacks, it marked the end of the clan period. They became members of society. They could no longer be called mountaineers and backwoodsmen.

The Blacks settled first in Winchester, in Scott County, Illinois, where they bought one hundred and sixty acres. In 1845, William Black sold this land, and he purchased two hundred acres in Cass County, near the village of Princeton, Illinois, on May 10, 1845. This land contained a large number of walnut trees of which the cabinetmaker could well make use.

Four boys were born into the Black family in Tennessee. In Scott county, Illinois, they had three boys and one girl. The first child born in Illinois—the fifth child in the family—was a boy, Greene Vardiman Black. He was born on August 3, 1836 (Fig. 8).

A Definite Purpose

From the beginning of their migration from Tennessee to Illinois, through their move from Scott County to their final home in Cass County (Figs. 9, 10), the Blacks had a definite, settled purpose: to establish a home in the fullest sense of the word in order to secure for their children the greatest measure of education and preparation for successful careers which their restricted information and limited financial means could afford.**

*Black and Black, p. 14
**Ibid., p. 28

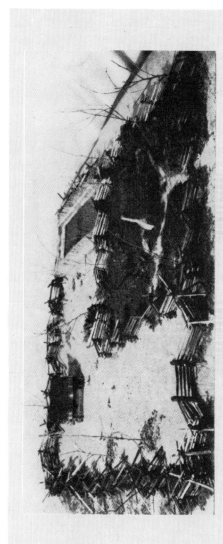

COTTAGE WHERE GREENE V. BLACK WAS BORN, AUGUST 3, 1836, IN SCOTT COUNTY, ILLINOIS.

Replica built from written description by Wm. L. Black of Virginia, Illinois, and verbal description by Judge J. M. Riggs of Winchester, Ill.

Figure 8

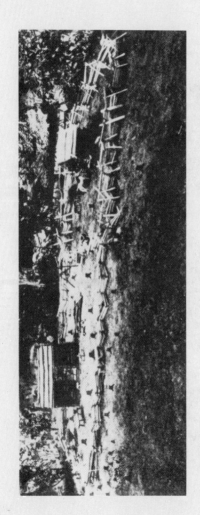

CABIN WHERE GREENE V. BLACK SPENT HIS CHILDHOOD IN CASS COUNTY, ILLINOIS.

Replica built from verbal descriptions.

Figure 9

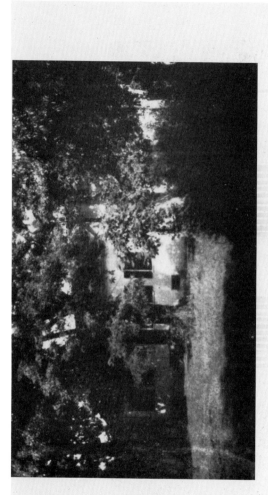

HOME WHERE GREENE V. BLACK SPENT HIS BOYHOOD, CASS COUNTY, ILLINOIS

Figure 10

The Black Family

Of G. V. Black's brothers, Thomas, the oldest (Fig. 11), went to college, where he studied medicine. Later, he became a widely known and highly respected practicing physician in Clayton, then a town in western Illinois. Thomas Black was elected to service in the Illinois legislature several times, and he rose to the rank of Colonel during the Civil War. Joseph, the second brother, was an architect, inventor, and builder. William, the third brother, and financier of the family, was first a farmer who changed his occupation and eventually became the president of an important bank. He held this post until the great age of ninety. The fourth older brother, Richmond, became the first blacksmith west of the Missouri River. G. V. Black's first younger brother, James, went to college in Pennsylvania. Later, he taught mathematics, became a Captain in the Army during the Civil War, and he was a rather famous portrait artist as well. Eventually he made banking his career. John, the youngest brother, went to school in Pennsylvania, and chose merchandising as his career. Jennie, the only daughter of the Black family, was sent to the Campbellite Church College for girls, and she later married a prosperous farmer.[*]

Pioneer Life

Hunting and fishing provided the most popular of the practical and helpful diversions of the pioneer family. Also, there were logrollings, house-raisings, cider-makings, and threshings, all of which were always

[*]Ibid., p. 27

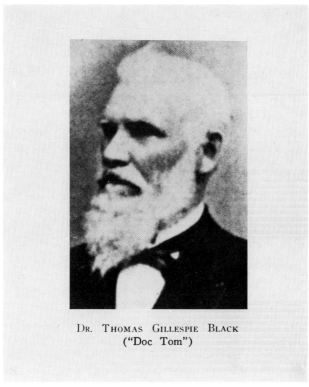

Dr. Thomas Gillespie Black
("Doc Tom")

Figure 11

accompanied by good dinners. There was music and dancing as well, and there were family and neighborhood singing parties.

On the more serious side, William Black valued education. He gave land for a school site, and he served as a school director of the Walnut School.

The pioneer credo consisted of only two parts: work and religion.

Parental Characteristics

William Black had a trade. He was a cabinetmaker. He was also a master of penmanship, a practical financier, and a deeply religious man who knew the Bible thoroughly to the extent that he could—and did—quote it at length, especially when he was called upon to lead the service of worship in the Campbellite Church.[*]

The little library which William Black had accumulated did not contain any novels. In fact, it is said that the modern novel of his day never invaded the family circle. William Black believed that there were enough good stories in the Bible to satisfy anybody.

William Black associated with the best people in the various communities where he lived. In addition to all that he did to provide the best that he could afford for the well-being of his family, he taught all of his sons the art of using tools. In this art, his son Greene Vardiman far surpassed the performances of the others.[**]

This, then, was the background; these were the roots of G. V. Black.

But what of G. V. Black himself?

In his boyhood, Greene Vardiman Black regarded going to the little log cabin school, with its slow methods of instruction, as a waste of time. Instead, he preferred hunting, fishing, and roaming the woods. He said he could learn more in the woods and among the neighbors in an hour than he could learn in school in a week.[***] Wild animals and all of nature were of real interest to him. Also, it has been written:

"He would not work on the farm. He was sent out to

[*]Ibid., p. 51
[**]Ibid., pp. 32, 59
[***]Ibid., p. 43

plow one afternoon. He plowed across the field to some willows, spent the afternoon studying plants, animals, and birds and then plowed a row back."* Much more existed to be learned in observing nature than in the slow routine of school and farm work—he doubtless thought.**

Considering the special importance of farm work to the pioneer family, his attitude left his pioneer parents puzzled. However, he was even-tempered—not ill-humored. He was an active person, actively interested in the world about him. He loved music, played the double-bass-viol, the flute, and the violin. He loved to take part in family singing.***

Fortunately, G. V. Black's mother was the one member of the family who understood him. Mary Vaughn Black is described as a woman who was very happy with her marriage to William Black and who was a perfect housewife and homemaker who possessed an unusual ability to understand and manage people.

While Mary Black understood her son and knew that he had ability, she was not certain just how this ability should be directed and developed. It was to her oldest son, Dr. Thomas Gillespie Black, that she would turn.

Choosing a Profession

In 1852, after seventeen years on the farm, G. V. Black went to live with his oldest brother, Thomas, who had graduated from Louisville Medical College in Kentucky and who was now a practicing physician in Clayton, Illinois. Dr. Thomas Black had a lucrative practice. In

*Schewe, p. 17
**Black and Black, pp. 47-48
***Ibid., pp. 46-48

order to help support himself at this time G. V. Black worked in a store and clerked in the post office.

"Doc Tom," as he was called, had a plan that "G. V." would read medicine under his direction. G. V. Black began the study of medicine, and it was said that perhaps he would have followed a medical career had not two things happened:

First, G. V. Black met and fell in love with Jane Coughenour whom he married, and then he met Dr. J. C. Speer, who was a dentist from the neighboring town of Mount Sterling, Illinois.

The net result of these two events was that he gave up the study of medicine temporarily and took up what was then described as the obscure trade of dentistry.

Operative Dentistry in the 19th Century

The oldest known book which discusses the cause of dental caries is the Artzney Buchlein written in the German language by an unknown author in 1530 (Fig. 12). Dr. Black translated one of this book's most remarkable statements as follows:

"Caries is a disease and evil of the teeth in which they become full of holes and hollow, which most often affects the back teeth; especially so when they are not cleaned of clinging particles of food which decompose, producing an acid moisture (literally, a sharp moisture) which eats them away and destroys them so that finally with much pain they rot away little by little" (Fig. 13).

Fig. 12 The first book to present a rational theory of the cause of dental caries was published by Michael Blum, of Leipzig, in 1530. The name of the author is not known.

Artzney Buch=
lein/wider allerlei kran=
ckeyten vnd gebrechen der zcen/gezogen
auß dem Galeno/Auicenna/Mesue/
Cornelio Celso vnd andern mehr
der Artzney Doctorn /seher
nützlich zu
lesen.
M. D. XXX.

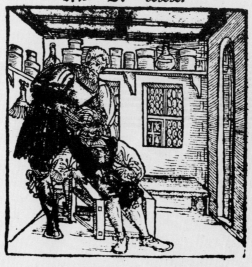

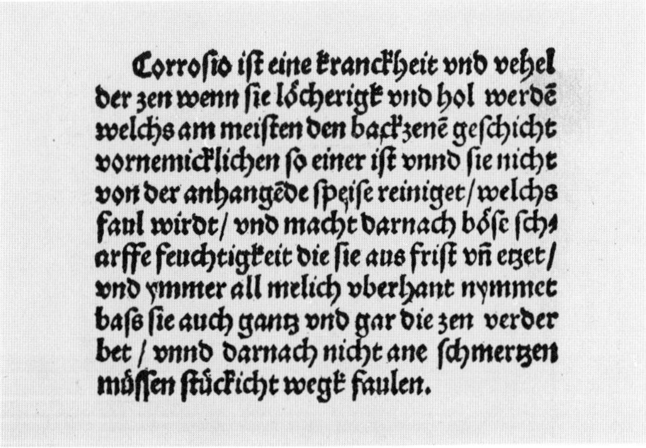

Corrosio ist eine kranckheit vnd vehel der zen wenn sie löcherigk vnd hol werdē welchs am meisten den backzenē geschicht vornemicklichen so einer ist vnnd sie nicht von der anhangēde speise reiniget/welchs faul wirdt/ vnd macht darnach böse scharffe feuchtigkeit die sie aus frist vñ etzet/ vnd ymmer all melich vberhant nymmet baß sie auch gantz vnd gar die zen verder bet / vnnd darnach nicht ane schmertzen müssen stückicht wegk faulen.

Fig. 13 Black translated this remarkable passage describing a theory of dental caries from the "Artzney-Buch" for his own "Pathology of the Hard Tissues of the Teeth," 1908.

Pierre Fauchard wrote his famous "Le Chirurgien Dentiste" which was published in Paris in 1728.
One of the best-known and most popular 19th century American textbooks on the practice of dentistry was The Principles and Practice of Dentistry by Chapin A. Harris. The first edition of Harris' book was published in Philadelphia in 1839 (Fig. 14). This book went through thirteen editions, the last of which appeared in 1896. Of this book's contribution to the advancement of the

Fig. 14 Title page of the first issue of the first American dental journal.

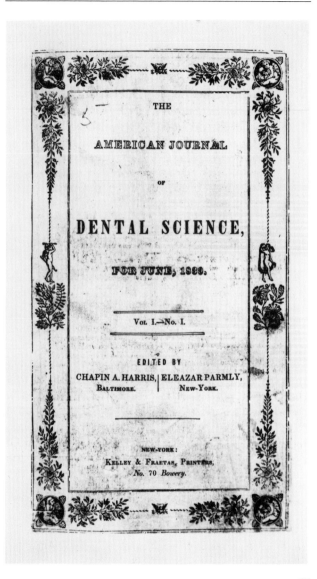

THE

AMERICAN JOURNAL

OF

DENTAL SCIENCE,

FOR JUNE, 1839.

VOL. I.—No. I.

EDITED BY

CHAPIN A. HARRIS, | ELEAZAR PARMLY,
BALTIMORE. | NEW-YORK.

NEW-YORK:
KELLEY & FRAETAS, PRINTERS,
No. 70 Bowery.

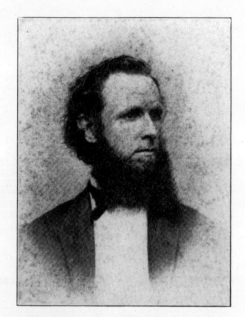

**Photograph of Dr. Black taken about 1865.
The Dental Review.**

Fig. 15   Photograph of G. V. Black published in *Dental Review*, vol. 24, 1910.

dental profession, G. V. Black was later to write in *The Dental Review* of 1892 (Fig. 15):
"It is a book that has descended to us from a past age and has been patched out time and again . . . The original was a splendid work and it bore good fruit. But

oh, the dust of the ages have gathered on its pages now. I know of no other book that has run such a gauntlet of revision and lived. This could not be but for the wonderful vitality of the original work and the reverence of the dental profession for the author."

Few illustrations of the desired outline form of cavity preparations are given in Harris' book or in any other 19th century book devoted either to operative dentistry or to the practice of dentistry in general. Most dental books of this period speak merely of the removal of the decay and of the placement of the restoration in the remaining space. This was the prevailing practice for treating dental caries in the middle of the 19th century. Some illustrations of cavity preparations from the dental periodical literature and the operative dentistry sections of the early dental textbooks are included in Figure 16. In most of the illustrations, the outline form extension of the cavity preparations falls far short of including the grooves and the pits—the weak points of the occlusal surfaces.

Two hundred and thirty-six years passed between John Josselyn's statement of the American dental problem before G. V. Black was to formulate the first scientific theoretical and practical attack on the American dental problem. With these passing years the labors and contributions of many dedicated people, including Fauchard, Hayden, and Harris in dentistry, and Pasteur, Koch, Lister, and Virchow in the basic sciences, along with many others, would be made and recorded.

In the past, when confronted with a problem of a microbiological and medical nature, man was often dimly aware of both the nature and the solution of the problem with which he was confronted. In other words,

Zum dritten das man die ausholung
wegk nimmet/welchs auch auf zweyerley
weyse geschicht/ Zum ersten das man das
loch vnd die aussfressunge mit einem subs
tilen meisselchen aber messerchen walchẽ/
aber mit einem andern instrument darzu
bequemicklich/wegk schabe/vnd reinige/
als dy practickanten wol wissen/vnd dar
zu erhaldung des andern teyles des zanes
das löchlichen mit golt blettern zu fullet.
Zum andern das mann gebrauche erytey
darzu dinlich welchs geschict mit Galles
epffel vnd wilder galgen so der zan nach
der reinigung darmit wirdt gefüllet.

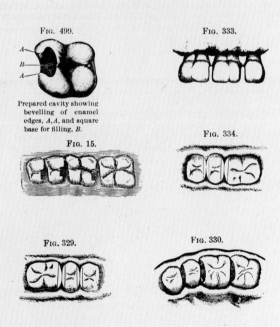

Fig. 499.

A
B
A

Prepared cavity showing
bevelling of enamel
edges, A, A, and square
base for filling, B.

Fig. 333.

Fig. 15.

Fig. 334.

Fig. 329.

Fig. 330.

initially man proceeded by intuition toward the solution to his problem. Later, however, when he developed theoretical knowledge—concepts by postulation—about the problem, in a relatively short period of time he achieved a lasting solution to the microbiological and medical problems with which he was confronted. *

Character Building

It is said that Thomas Black, who was the original source of G. V. Black's professional ideals, must have been disappointed, but that G. V. Black never allowed himself to have a falling-out with anyone.** Nonetheless, even as a youth, he preferred his own methods of self-education to the traditional methods of education which he would not follow.

*Dubos, pp. 71-72; 114-116
**Black and Black, p. 62

Fig. 16   Black's translation: "In the third plan, the hollow place is done away with (taken away—removed) which is done in one of two ways. First, the soft part of the cavity and the decayed part is cut away with small chisels, knives, files or other suitable instruments, and cleaned, as is well known to practitioners. Then for the saving of the remaining parts of the tooth, the cavity is filled with gold leaf. Otherwise one may use a suitable gum prepared with nutgalls and hyssop to fill the cavity after cleaning it. (From "A Work on Operative Dentistry," vol. I, Medico-Dental Publ. Co., Chicago, 1908) Also pictured are outline forms of cavity preparations typical of dental periodical and textbook literature of the 19th century. Most of the central fissures and the pits of the occlusal surfaces are not included in the outline form of the cavity preparations.

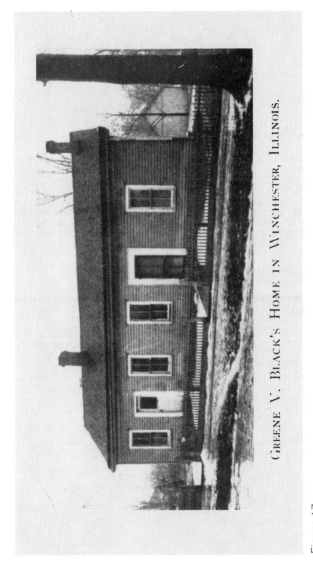

GREENE V. BLACK'S HOME IN WINCHESTER, ILLINOIS.

Figure 17

After spending a few weeks with Dr. Speer, G. V. Black felt that he had learned all that he could. So, in 1857, he began the practice of dentistry with an office in Winchester, Illinois, and an itinerant practice in neighboring towns, thus becoming the first dentist in Scott County (Fig. 17).

What characteristics did G. V. Black possess which enabled him to begin the solo practice of dentistry so soon, after such a short association with Dr. Speer? The following traits have been suggested:

A natural aptitude for gathering facts, studious disposition, constant perseverance, sustained interest, manual dexterity, power of observation, ability to make correct deductions, determination, and above all, the power of forethoughtful concentration.*

Study of Basic Sciences

G. V. Black would continue the medical studies which he began under the direction of his brother Dr. Thomas Black, and he would make these studies a life-long habit. Black worked diligently to learn all that he could about the newly developing science of bacteriology. He studied the deductively formulated scientific works of Pasteur, Koch, Loeb, Erlich, Colin, Schwaan, Lister, Virchow, (Fig. 18) and many others. Lister had revolutionized surgery with new methods of applied asepsis and antisepsis, and Virchow had written *Cellular Pathology.*

Black taught himself German, Latin, and French so that he could read many of these authors in their original languages. Thus he was able to study all of the available information on any subject in which he was inter-

*Ibid., p. 341

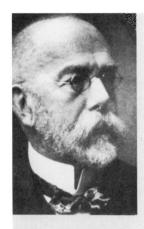

ROBERT KOCH

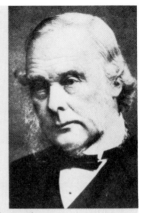

JOSEPH LISTER, 1827–1912

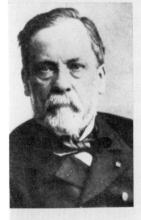

LOUIS PASTEUR, 1822–1897

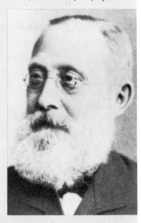

RUDOLPH VIRCHOW, 1821–1902

ested. He read *Cellular Pathology* in the original German and in the English translation and was inspired by it. He also studied algebra, geometry, and the basic sciences in his own way.*

Because jewelers as well as dentists had a common interest in the physical properties of precious metals, Black quickly became friends with the jewelers of Winchester. He also visited the clockmaker and was himself a skilled worker in brass and other metals.

Frederick B. Noyes, a contemporary of G. V. Black, in Vol. 30 of *The Dental Review* would write:

"There are certain qualities of mind that must be present to make one great in science. The first of these is patience: patience to compile the facts; patience to spend days, weeks, months, years if necessary, to fill out the series of observations, and follow out the necessary relationships; patience to meet defeat by seeking its cause and eliminating one cause of failure after another. The second necessary quality is accuracy of observation; the ability to note conditions exactly to the minutest detail, without prejudice or the predetermined seeking for certain anticipated results. Thirdly is

*Ibid., pp. 145, 348

Fig. 18   Black studied the works of these men, among others, and was inspired by them. All of these great scientists had a strong interest in the study of nature for the purpose of furthering the health of the public. Their shared characteristics included iron wills, equanimity and persistence in the face of scientific obstacles, love of research for its own sake and for its contributions to progress, and "creative ignoring" of opposition to the introduction of new ideas.

47

needed a logical faculty: the ability to reason correctly from the observed facts, to give each fact its proper weight and significance, and discover the relationship of cause and effect. The final quality, and most important of all, is a clear and true imagination: the ability to picture the unseen, to discover the significance of apparently unimportant observations, to catch the real meaning in a series of observations; the seeing of the unseen before it becomes real—this is the greatest qualification of all. That man becomes great in scientific fields who, viewing a series of observed facts, sees them drop into a sequence and order, his mind bridging the gaps so that he goes to work to fill in the spaces, until the sequence, instead of a partial one, becomes complete, and a great general principle is discovered. I have sometimes thought that one reason why America has become so prominent in original scientific investigations in the last few years, was partly due to the recent frontier training of the American people. The conditions of frontier life made necessary, closeness of observation, and the correct interpretation or reasoning from the conditions observed. Life itself often depended on noting the footprint in the grass and recognizing it as made by friend or foe. All of the tricks of woodcraft are based upon correct reasoning from accurate observation."

Thus, from his early beginning with the relationship of direct experience and observation of nature, G. V. Black eventually arrived at a new relationship to nature through the study of deductively formulated science.*

*Northrop (b), chapts. 4 and 6

Chapter 3

Community

Over the long span of his active life, G. V. Black was a man who related himself to other people through service to the community in which he lived.

Life for G. V. Black as a young dentist in the town of Winchester, Illinois (Fig. 19), was happy and successful, both professionally and domestically.

His happiness was not to last, however, for the Civil War began and G. V. Black enlisted in the Union Army.

While he was in the service, he suffered a knee injury which terminated his military career and which also required a long period of recuperation in the hospital in Louisville, Kentucky.

When he started to feel better—but was not yet well enough to move—he began his recovery. He did three things. He read the Bible through three times. He devoted himself to training his left hand to be as useful as his right. Now he could write two letters home at the same time. This newly acquired ambidexterity would come in handy in the future practice of dentistry. Finally, he observed and studied physicians and their ways.

Tragedy and Grief

The Black's first child died, and a second child, Carl, was born during this time. Then tragedy struck again when his wife was stricken with tuberculosis and died in 1863.

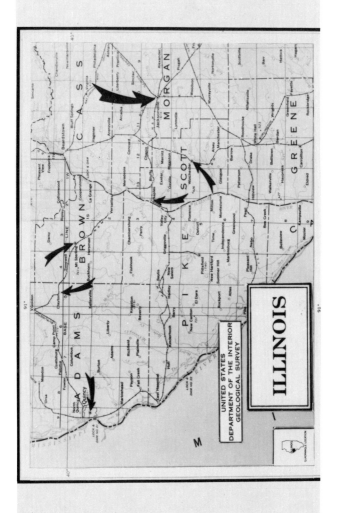

For G. V. Black, temporarily, the joy of living had disappeared. The normal course of his life had been interrupted by unexpected, undesired events. First, the war brought injury and hospitalization; next came the death of his child, and finally, there was—what might well have seemed to have been the last straw—the death of his wife. It seemed that his life and all of his plans for the future had been crushed. G. V. Black, however, was not one to fall prey to the evils of an obvious or an insidious self-pity, or a lack of faith.

New plans, therefore, would have to be made. His young son Carl was taken to the home of the grandparents Black and was looked after there. To G. V. Black, his father's house was always as a safe and friendly port—it was a haven which was a great source of comfort and strength, especially in a stormy time of crisis.*

Move to Jacksonville

Black had to break up his home in Winchester as he was not able to continue his life and work there due to the unhappy memories of all that had happened during the war. He chose to move to Jacksonville, Illinois, a city of 10,000 inhabitants and of academies, colleges, and state institutions; there were seventeen literary and scientific societies as well and all of this in a forest

*Black and Black, pp. 62, 103

Fig. 19   Arrows on the map indicate places important in G. V. Black's life which are mentioned in the text.

setting. The setting stimulated memories of his earlier days. Jacksonville was a place which was richly endowed with streams and a variety of trees: oak, maple, and the enduring walnut—a tree which was for him a symbol of a long life, security, and protection. There he would start practice again, in 1863.*

In Jacksonville, G. V. Black began practice in partnership with a Dr. J. C. Cox, who soon retired. Black bought out Cox and thus realized the main objective of his move to Jacksonville: to secure a better business opportunity (Fig. 20).**

Now he began to take an active and leading part in the life of the community. Here, at this period, he met Miss Elizabeth Akers Davenport who had been a student at the Jacksonville Female Academy. On September 14, 1865, they were married (Fig. 21).

Family Life and a Demanding Schedule

Black brought his young son Carl to his new situation. It was said that:

"No man ever made a happier choice in marriage, for Elizabeth Black was an exceptional woman of refined manners, pleasing personality and gentle dignity, who, with rare insight, tact and devotion, filled a place in the life of her gifted husband. With ardor she entered into his scientific ambitions, and was proud of his many achievements."*** More children followed; the Black family grew.

At about this time, as he continued his studies, G. V. Black worked on a demanding schedule. He began his

*Ibid., p. 112
**Ibid., p. 107
***Anon., p. 18

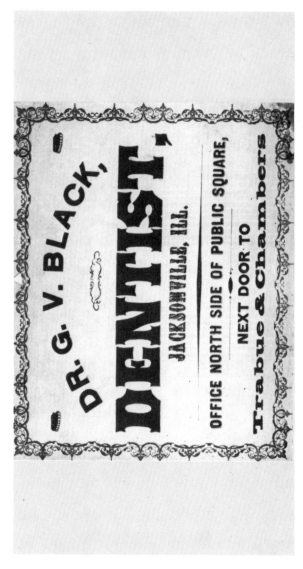

Fig. 20   Black's first dental office sign, in Jacksonville, Illinois.

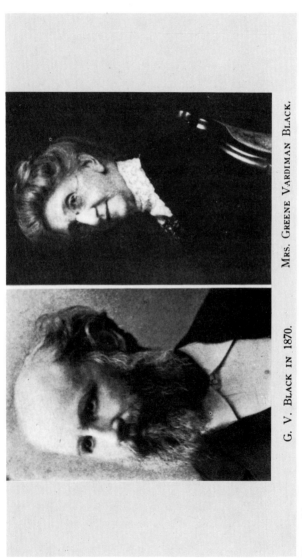

MRS. GREENE VARDIMAN BLACK.

G. V. BLACK IN 1870.

Figure 21

daily private practice of dentistry in his office at nine o'clock and worked until noon. After lunch, he worked from one-thirty to five o'clock. He then left his office and went home to dinner (Fig. 22).

When dinner was finished, he made it his habit to spend two hours, from six to eight o'clock, with his family. This time was most often spent with music and family singing. With regard to music, it must be noted well that Dr. Black was no mere dilettante. He was capable of performing Schubert's Serenade on the violin, and all of the favorite songs of the time. His daughters often provided the vocal and piano accompaniment. Friends who visited his home in the evening were frequently treated to such a Black family concert.[*]

When this family time was over, Mrs. Black was very skilled at whisking the children away from their father so that they would not bother him. G. V. Black would then turn to his scientific studies and research, at which he would work until roughly one, or even three o'clock in the morning.[**] Black once told Dr. Frederick Noyes that in other years he had formed the habit of giving the hours from five to six in the morning to his scientific studies. He would try to thoroughly exhaust the subject under study before beginning the study of another subject.

[*]Dunning, p. 414
[**]Black and Black, p. 183

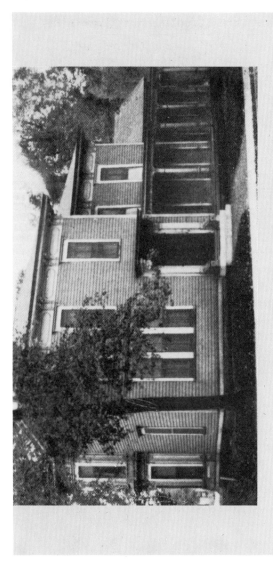

G. V. BLACK'S HOME, 1865-1898 AND OFFICE, 1876-1898, JACKSONVILLE, ILLINOIS.

Figure 22

Thomas Gilmer: Surgeon, Sailor, Friend

At the banquet of the Chicago Odontographic Society, in 1910, Dr. Thomas Gilmer told of his first meeting with G. V. Black. He said:

"After locating in Waverly, it was not long before I came in contact with Dr. Black's patients. . . . I saw beautiful restorations; I saw beautifully contoured fillings, artistically finished, perfectly polished, and I also saw exemplified in the mouths of his patients even at that early day that which has since become a byword the world over—'extension for prevention.' "*

The first time Dr. Gilmer visited G. V. Black's office in Jacksonville, he noted: "I saw all sorts of things, a big foot turning lathe, fine tools of all kinds, an anvil and things that go with it, mechanical drawings on the walls"** (Fig. 23).

Dr. Gilmer continued his remarks:

"About 1878, I found Dr. Black busily engaged in the study of bacteriology and laying the foundation for his great work, 'Formation of Poisons by Microorganisms.' He was always at work on some problem, not always of a professional nature, but all sorts of problems. I have never known a man so prolific. He can do more things and do them well, than anyone I have ever known. He also completed his medical education about this time, went before the State Medical Board, passed a most rigid examination and was licensed to practice medicine. During this time, he almost overdid the matter of study. He worked at the chair all day and with his books and microscope at night. He grew so thin that his friends remonstrated with him, but it did no good, work

*Anon. pp. 114-115
**Ibid., pp. 116-120

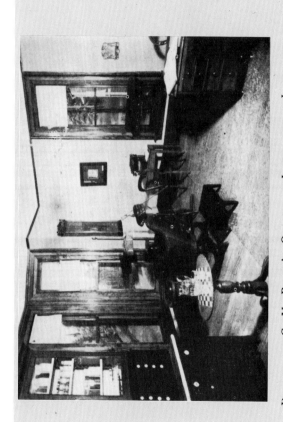

REPLICA OF G. V. BLACK'S OFFICE IN JACKSONVILLE, ILLINOIS, IN THE G. V. BLACK MEMORIAL ROOMS AT NORTHWESTERN UNIVERSITY DENTAL SCHOOL.

he would, the habit was so fixed, he could not stop it. "During Dr. Black's time of poor health, I persuaded him to come over to Quincy, and spend a few days with me. I was always a water dog. I used to sail much. Early Sunday morning we went down to the river and I got the Doctor into my sailboat and up the river we went. When I showed him how to manage the sheets and the rudder, I suggested that he take the boat, which he did. We sailed all that day and when we got back, he could give me pointers in sailing, so apt was he in learning."

Gilmer went on to relate the conversation which took place when he told G. V. Black that he had developed a surgical practice and was treating a large number of fractures of the jaws. Gilmer's account of the conversation went as follows:

"I told the Doctor about these, when he said, 'You must write a paper for the Illinois State Dental Society on fractures.' I said, 'Unless I have illustrations, such a paper will not be well received.' He said, 'You write the paper and I will illustrate it.' So I prepared the paper and took it over to him. We went over it and agreed on what was necessary to illustrate it. He set to work and after a time wrote me. 'The pictures are ready, come over and see what you think of them.' You may imagine my surprise to find that this busy man had found time to make forty life-size water colors for me, illustrating every part of my paper (Fig. 24). The pictures were so fine that it made me feel that the paper was not good enough to go with them. I rewrote the paper several

Fig. 23   The replica of G. V. Black's office is an exhibit in the collection of the Smithsonian Institution, Washington, D.C.

88   Illinois State Dental Society.

FIG. 27.

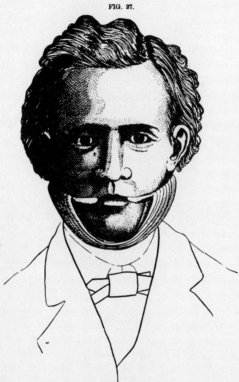

Side arm interdental Splint applied. A gutta percha or plaster paris boot may be used on the chin.

times, trying to bring it up to the pictures, but I fear I never succeeded. Those pictures today are the best and really the only complete set of good illustrations on the subject. They were copied in dental journals all over the world."*

Dental Literature and Dental Society

In 1867, G. V. Black began to write a series of popular articles about dentistry in the local newspaper, the *Jacksonville Journal.*

When the Missouri State Dental Association had held its first meeting, in June of the year preceding the appearance of the series of articles on dentistry in the *Jacksonville Journal,* G. V. Black had become a member of this dental association.

Black usually induced one or more of his local colleagues to go with him to the State Dental Society meetings. He always maintained excellent personal relationships with his fellow dentists. He was thirty-four years old when he was elected president of the Illinois

*Ibid., pp. 119-124

Fig. 24   One of Black's 40 illustrations for Thomas L. Gilmer's article on fractures of the mandible, published in *Transactions of the Illinois State Dental Society* (page 88, 1881). Gilmer later noted: "Dr. Black had a wonderful faculty for drawing. Once, when visiting him in Jacksonville, thirty years ago, I found him writing the specifications for a business house, the architectural and working drawings having been made in every detail by himself. That building still stands on the south side of the public square in Jacksonville and is in keeping architecturally with others more modern." (*Dental Review,* 1916)

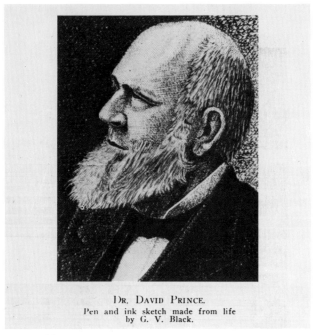

DR. DAVID PRINCE.
Pen and ink sketch made from life
by G. V. Black.

Figure 25a

State Dental Society.* G. V. Black also became a member of the local medical society.

Dr. David Prince (Fig. 25a), a surgeon, whom Black often assisted in operations, influenced him to study pathology. They studied pathology as taught by Virchow. It was from this study that he saw the need to study the normal. He made thousands of slides and a large case (Fig. 25b).

*Black and Black, pp. 139-140

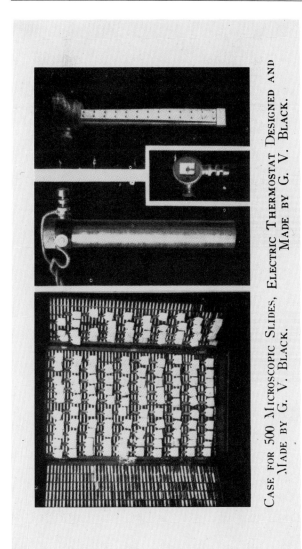

CASE FOR 500 MICROSCOPIC SLIDES, ELECTRIC THERMOSTAT DESIGNED AND MADE BY G. V. BLACK.

CASE FOR 500 MICROSCOPIC SLIDES, MADE BY G. V. BLACK.

Figure 25b

If he needed any type of mechanical equipment, the most common way for him to get it was to make it himself—dental items and others.

In 1868, he was studying chemistry. This study enabled him to manufacture his own "laughing gas." Another outgrowth of his interest in chemistry was that chemistry classes for the community were begun and were held in Dr. Black's office. Dr. Black was selected to be the teacher, and both men and women from the community of Jacksonville attended these classes.*

Two years later, in 1870, G. V. Black designed, patented, and manufactured the cord-driven, foot-powered dental engine.** He also designed many dental research instruments such as the gnathodynamometer, the phagodynamometer, the manudynamometer, the amalgam micrometer, and others. He constructed many of these instruments himself.

"One of the most interesting mechanical gadgets was a patent, repeating rat-trap. When he moved into the home he bought in Jacksonville it was infested with rats and he set about to clear them out. With a big, heavy clock spring as a basis, he devised a repeating machine. Careful measurements were made of a rat's head and the "contraption" was so arranged that when the rat pulled the bait the spring was released and a sharp pin struck the rat in the head, piercing the skull and knocking the rat across the room. The next morning he found a pile of six to a dozen rats catapulted to the opposite corner of the room."***

*Ibid., pp. 121, 134
**Dunning, p. 411
***Black and Black. p. 131

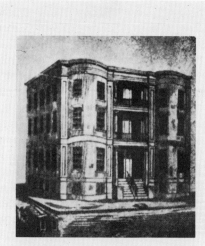

THE MISSOURI DENTAL COLLEGE
WHERE G. V. BLACK TAUGHT
1870 to 1880.

Figure 26

Dental Education

When the Missouri College was chartered on September 15, 1866, G. V. Black was one of its trustees (Fig. 26). He served on its faculty from 1870 to 1881. He lectured on pathology. His lectures were never repetitious from year to year and were constantly kept up-to-date.[*]

In 1878, registration and licensing of dentists began. As he had many years of experience in practicing

[*]Ibid, pp. 169-170

dentistry, he could have made direct application for a license, but he elected to take the examination. The passing grade was eighty percent, and thirty-four candidates took this examination. Needless to say, he was among the seventeen who passed, and he received his license certificate on January 15, 1878.

Dr. Black was elected in 1881 to be the first president of the Illinois State Board of Dental Examiners, which office he held until 1887.

In 1886, he was teaching at the Chicago College of Dental Surgery. In addition to a busy private practice and his lecture series at the dental school, he had also prepared and delivered or published twenty-four papers—an average of two papers per month.

G. V. Black's method of writing has been described as follows:

The facts were persistently and laboriously searched-out and were then recorded in painstaking detail; the search for facts was fairly exhausted; experiments and observations were always made at least three times; the facts were assembled and classified; and the deductions and the conclusion were written. He was a master of painstaking detail. He never concentrated on how quickly he could work but rather on the quality of his work. His high level of productivity was the result of his unremitting study and industry. There was no waste of time. While G. V. Black always seemed to be working on papers and although his scientific output was immense, it has been noted that "he never confined his activities entirely to the dental art. He always kept himself posted on what was going on in the world. He was not a 'scientific hermit.'"[*]

*Ibid., p. 152

Community Life

G. V. Black continued to take an active part in the community life of Jacksonville (Fig. 27). He was a member of the Campbellite Church - the church of his father and mother - and he never left it. He was president of the Third Ward Republican Club, and he was a member of the I.O.O.F. Library Association. He sang in the choir of the Jacksonville Philharmonic Society and was a master of his Masonic Lodge, in which he stayed active until 1878. On October 30, 1887, Dr. G. V. Black was elected a "correspondent" of the Academy of Natural Sciences of Philadelphia, Pennsylvania.

Before the Jacksonville Literary Union, which met, regardless of the weather, every Monday evening in the homes of its members, Dr. Black read a paper in 1878 about the need for a paid fire department in Jacksonville. Some of the titles of his other nondental papers were "Water, Water, Water," "Sam Marsden's Race for Life, Story of the Illinois Prairies," and "Out Sailing." Most of these papers originally were deposited in the Jacksonville Literary Union and are now in the collection of the library of the Dental School of Northwestern University. The Jacksonville Literary Union - valued for its own sake, indeed! - must have also provided a powerful creative stimulus to G. V. Black's professional work in dentistry (Fig. 28).

Dr. Black was an active member of the Jacksonville Literary Union from 1873 to 1897 when he became an honorary member of this remarkable society which was founded in 1863 and is still in existence.[*]

The first bicycle had appeared in England back in

[*]Mrs. Carl E. Black, II

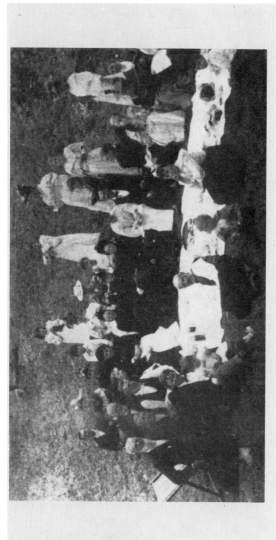

G. V. BLACK AT FAMILY PICNIC, WALNUT GROVE FARM.

Figure 27

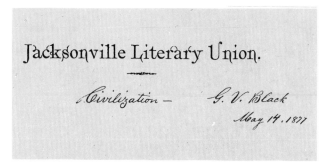

Fig. 28 Title page of one of the G. V. Black non-dental papers deposited in the Jacksonville Literary Union. Black took quiet pride in his 20-year record of perfect attendance at Monday night meetings of the group, which he valued highly.

1867. Dr. Black owned the first bicycle in his region - homemade, of course. The wheels were almost buggy wheels with iron tires. A machinist fashioned the framework, handle, and handlebars; the device had a movable seat. Black became famous for his "night rides" when he would visit such places as the newspaper office, the police station, and the waterworks. These rides were for him relaxation from his rigorous daily schedule in one sense, and an expression of his interest in the well-being and problems of the community in another.*

Black informed his children that during this time, until the year of 1880, he had long dark hair, and at one time, he had a full beard which reached down to his beltline, together with a moustache which could be placed back over his ears.**

*Black and Black, pp. 155, 184
**Ibid., p. 133

The Black's home life was described as being ideal in every respect. Before meals, a humble grace with thanks for God's blessing and mercy was always said by G. V. Black.

Dr. Thomas Gilmer, G. V. Black's good friend and a frequent visitor to the Black's home, wrote:

"At the dinner table, scientific matters were dropped, and we just had a good time with the family and general conversation."[*]

"G. V. Black was the model father and husband in the family circle, the ideal professional man in public life, and the scholar and scientist who labored in solitude and without fanfare. Despite the large amount of time and money he spent in extensive research, which has immeasurably enriched dentistry, he never neglected his practice, and always derived sufficient income therefrom to provide for his family, giving his children every educational advantage, and to leave enough at his death to provide for his dependents."[**]

G. V. Black's son, Dr. Carl Ellsworth Black, was a surgeon and co-author of the book, From Pioneer to Scientist, a biography of Dr. G. V. Black and his other son, Dr. Arthur D. Black. Dr. Arthur D. Black, following his father and Dr. Thomas Gilmer, became Dean of The Dental School of Northwestern University and was the Compiler of the "Index of the Periodical Dental Literature," forerunner of today's "Index to Dental Literature."

Like his father and his older brother "Doc Tom" before him, G. V. Black related himself actively and wholeheartedly to other people through service to the community in which he lived.

[*]Ibid., p. 121
[**]Schewe, pp. 18-19

Chapter 4

Purpose

Dr. Greene Vardiman ("G. V.") Black had become a man of overarching purpose. He was contributing the results of his life and labors toward the development of scientific modern dentistry (Fig. 29).

Dr. Greene Vardiman Black had become a man of - to use the word of Professor John E. Smith - "overarching" purpose.* In stressing the importance of this kind of purpose, Professor Smith writes:

"In pursuing a goal, most important is discovering *what counts* for the purpose at hand, as distinct from what does not count, as true and as well attested as it may be."**

Dr. Black had acquired the honorary D.D.S. degree from Missouri Dental College in 1877 and an M.D. degree from the Chicago Medical College (later Northwestern University) in 1884 (Fig. 30).

Later, he would receive three more honorary degrees: Sc.D., Illinois College, 1892; LL.D., Northwestern University, 1898; and Sc.D. from the University of Pennsylvania, 1915.

Microorganisms and Dental Caries

"In 1880, Pasteur had discovered the streptococcus and pneumococcus. Black immunized chickens against cholera—a new method in a new field. The

*Smith (a), p. 328
**Smith (b), p. 4

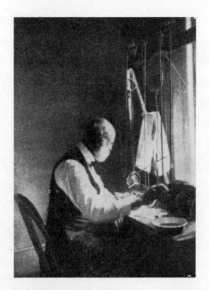

G. V. BLACK OPERATING HIS MACHINE FOR GRINDING MICROSCOPIC SECTIONS OF THE TEETH AND BONE IN HIS NORTHWESTERN DENTAL SCHOOL LABORATORY.

Figure 29

discoveries by Eberth in the cause of typhoid fever, Laveran in malaria, and Pasteur and Sternberg in the carrying of pneumonia organisms in the healthy mouth—all of these discoveries fired the mind of this dentist.*

*Schewe, p. 19

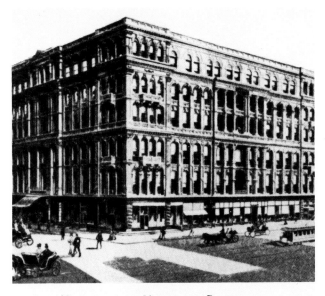

NORTHWESTERN UNIVERSITY BUILDING
The Dental School occupied the three top floors when
Dr. Greene V. Black became Dean.

Figure 30

In 1883, Black prepared his first book, "The Formation of Poisons by Microorganisms." This was an important book because therein:

"He was the first to announce that all life including microorganisms produces injurious waste products and that they are largely responsible for disease including dental caries." He quoted Virchow and discussed the works of Klebs, Volkmann, Beale, Pasteur, and Koch to show that microorganisms produce disease. He went to Germany and France to deliver lectures about the results of his research (Fig. 31).

"Periosteum and Peridental Membrane," G. V. Black's second book, was published in 1887. He prepared all of this book's sixty-seven hand-drawn illustrations from his own microscopic slides (Fig. 32).

Petoskey Interlude

"In 1887, Dr. Black had found it necessary to have a complete rest and change of occupation."* From 1865 to 1877, he had been at work on his self-taught fundamental and dental education. He had become deeply engrossed in bacteriology as a new science and in its application to medicine and dentistry as a cause of disease. Self-imposed investigation, familiarity with work in other countries and their languages, and the need to make all of his own apparatus and to learn bacteriological and microscopic techniques—all of this plus his regular professional work—caused his health to suffer badly under the strain.

A number of Jacksonville families had begun to spend their summer vacations in Petoskey, Michigan (Fig. 33), and in 1887 he spent several weeks at this place.

*Black and Black, p. 213

Fig. 31   Ten conclusions from Part 1 of the first edition of Black's first book, "The Formation of Poisons by Microorganisms," P. Blakiston, Son & Co., Philadelphia, 1884, pp. 74-76.

SUMMING UP.

Having passed in review, briefly, the rise and progress of the Germ Theory of Disease, we may sum up the principal points thus :—

1st. In the seventeenth and eighteenth centuries, intelligent observers of contagious diseases, after much study of the subject, came to the conclusion they were caused and propagated by a process identical with or similar to fermentation and decomposition.

2d. There was much study of the processes of fermentation and decomposition, in order to arrive at a more clear understanding of the causes of epidemic and contagious diseases with the view of prevention and cure. These experiments demonstrated that the fermentations and decompositions were something different from ordinary chemical phenomena.

3d. The yeast plant was discovered by Schwan and Latour, in 1838. These gentlemen announced distinctly that the chemical changes of vinous fermentation are caused by the life and growth of this plant. They disproved, by experiment, the previous hypothesis, that oxygen is the active agent in any of the similar processes ; and, reasoning from this discovery, came to the conclusion that all the fermentations, decompositions, miasms and contagions were caused by the life force.

4th. These conclusions were attacked by chemists, notably, by Professor Liebig, who denied both the facts claimed and the conclusions arrived at, since which time there has been a continuous discussion of the subject.

5th. In 1854, Schroeder conclusively disproved the existence of gaseous ferments claimed by chemists, by admitting air filtered through cotton batting to sterilized fluids without causing fermentation.

6th. From 1857 to 1861 Pasteur successfully worked out all the more ordinary fermentations by his fractional flask cultivations, and proved each of them to have a specific plant growth as its cause. He also showed that none of the decompositions could proceed without living organisms, though the specific organism belonging to each was not clearly made out.

7th. Basing his efforts on the results of the last two, Mr. Lister introduced his antiseptic treatment of wounds, in 1865, which has proved a panacea for most of the dreaded infectious wound troubles in all hospital surgical practice.

8th. M. Pasteur, Dr. Koch and others have succeeded in isolating a number of distinct disease-producing germs, and causing the specific diseases in animals, regularly, by planting these germs under the skin, and Dr. Koch, especially, has succeeded in doing this after freeing the organisms of all possible following of decomposing matter by growing them upon dry slides.

9th. This much having been proven, the continued observation of numerous other organisms of distinct form and character, always associated with specific forms of disease, warrants the inference that these diseases are also caused by specific organisms.

10th. All the foregoing taken together gives strong presumptive evidence that all contagious and infectious diseases are produced by disease germs.

Figure 31 (Continued)

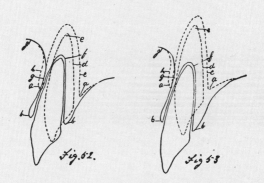

Figs. 52 and 53. Diagramatic illustration of the movement of a central incisor during the growth of the alveolar process between the age of twelve aud twenty-one years. The broken lines represent the tooth and its alveolus at twelve years of age, and the solid the same tooth at twenty-one.

Fig. 52 represents the minimum movement, while fig. 53 represents the maximum movement, as ordinarily observed. The figures are lettered alike. The growth of the process is represented by the movement from *a, a* to *b, b*. The tooth is carried forward with this growth, and the alveolus is filled with new bone from the line *c* to the line *f*.

Fig. 32   One of the 67 illustrations from Black's second book, "A Study of the Histological Characters of the Periosteum and Peridental Membrane," W. T. Keener, Chicago, 1887

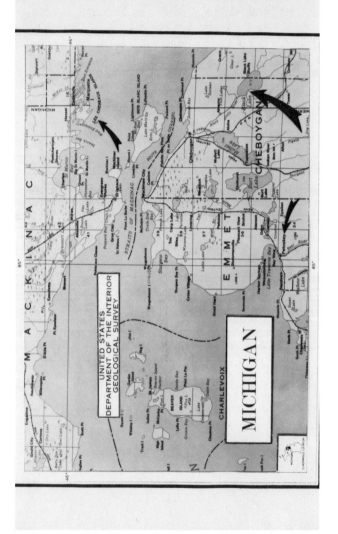

Black discovered that sailing on the lakes gave him the greatest rest and recreation and decided to obtain a boat of his own. He had his own ideas about boat design. He consulted boat builders, made drawings, and studied other boats. Finally, he planned and designed his own ideal boat which, when it was completed, he christened 'The Microbe.'

The selection of the name, 'The Microbe,' was in deference to the cause of the nervous strain which had forced Black's turn toward the North Country. Construction of this boat was accomplished during his second year in Northern Michigan.*

The key features of the boat's design were: starboard and port iceboards rather than centerboards, allowing the cockpit to be used for a bunk; watertight compartments fore and aft; the cockpit could be covered with waterproofed boards and made watertight; boom and gaff could be raised and propped at the end and then covered with canvas to make a tent which could serve as a complete camp on shore or at anchor. Two of the boards which covered the cockpit could be joined together and had legs so that they could serve as a table ashore. Just aft of the cockpit was a metal-lined well with a separate hatch which contained two oil stoves. She was eighteen feet long and four feet six on the beam and sloop-rigged.**

G. V. Black became a sailor and sailed all of the lakes of the region. In addition, he explored the terrain and became acquainted with the settlers of this region, and he wrote many of his non-dental papers on these vaca-

*Ibid., p. 213
**Ibid., p. 214

Figure 33

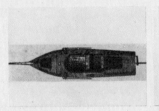
Pen and ink drawing of "The Microbe"
made by G. V. Black.

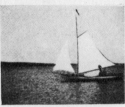
Sailing "The Microbe."

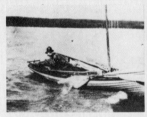
After running in through a heavy sea
from Lake Huron.

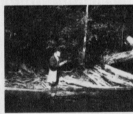
Trout fishing in northern Michigan.

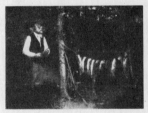
Ten black bass caught with one rod
in thirty minutes, in the Wisconsin
River, 1897.

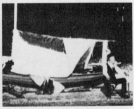
"The Microbe" camp.

tions. The vacations, both initially and later, were a healthy, active, sudden turning toward nature, as well as a refreshing change of activity, and the nondental writings perhaps provided an opportunity for self-training and practice in writing, as well as for relaxation. Thus did he revitalize himself—recharge his batteries, as it were—at this time, and he revisited Petoskey for fifteen years, each summer, thereafter (Fig. 34).

In 1890, the first edition of G. V. Black's third book, "Dental Anatomy" (Fig. 35), was published. Of this book, Dr. Fred Gethro has written:

"Practically every dental school in the country uses Dr. Black's 'Dental Anatomy.' He did this so well that nobody else has ever attempted to write a book on this subject."*

A New Epoch in Operative Dentistry

In the late 1880's, G. V. Black began work on a paper about the enamel margins of cavity preparations. It was a work which was to usher in a new epoch in the practice of operative dentistry.

As it was necessary for the dentist to be familiar with the normal histological structure of the tooth before

*Ibid., p. 238

Fig. 34   Scenes from the Petoskey Interlude. Black Lake, in northern Michigan, was named after G. V. Black (Black and Black, p. 215, see map of Michigan, Fig. 33). Black's outings on the water were of great benefit to him. He had a great reputation as a bold and daring sailor among the Indians and fishermen of the region (Gilmer).

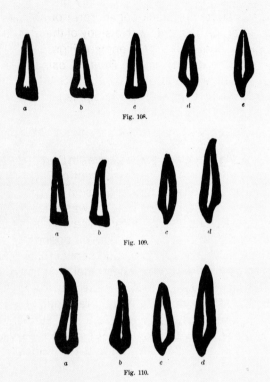

FIG. 108 * (Par. 160).—THE PULP CHAMBER OF THE UPPER CENTRAL INCISOR. a, b, Mesio-distal sections of the young teeth, showing the three short horns of the pulp; c, mesio-distal section of a tooth from an adult; d, e, labio-lingual sections.

FIG. 109 * (Par. 160).—PULP CHAMBER OF THE UPPER LATERAL INCISOR.—a, b, Mesio-distal sections; c, labio-lingual sections; d, labio-lingual section of a very long lateral incisor.

FIG. 110 * (Par. 163)—PULP CHAMBER OF THE UPPER CUSPIDS. a, b, Mesio-distal sections; c, d, labio-lingual sections.

* Illustration, actual size.

considering the pathological lesions of the enamel and dentin and their treatment by cavity preparation and dental restoration, Black began Part I of his five-part ground-breaking article with a study of the normal histological appearance of the enamel (Figs. 36-38). This article first appeared in *The Dental Cosmos,* vol. 33, 1891, which was published by the S. S. White Dental Manufacturing Company, Philadelphia.

'Extension for Prevention'

In 1891, Black published five articles in *Dental Cosmos* on the subject of "The Management of Enamel Margins," in which the phrase 'extension for prevention' first appeared in print. The phrase was to become the very cornerstone of scientific tooth cavity preparation. The heading with which G. V. Black opened the first section of Part 2 of "The Management of Enamel Margins" was "Weak Lines of the Enamel." In this section, Black illustrated and discussed the way in which developmental faults in the enamel predisposed teeth to caries of the enamel (Fig. 39).

The epoch-making title which G. V. Black gave to Section 2 of Part 2 of this paper was "Extension for Prevention, or Position of Enamel Margins considered

Fig. 35   Illustration from Black's third book, "Descriptive Anatomy of the Human Teeth," Wilmington Dental Manufacturing Co., Philadelphia, 1890. Here Black suggests that silhouettes which give the form of the tooth and pulp chamber can be made by inking the smooth, flat-ground longitudinal sections of extracted teeth on an inked pad and then impressing the inked surface on paper supported by a sheet of semi soft rubber (teeth shown 75% of original size).

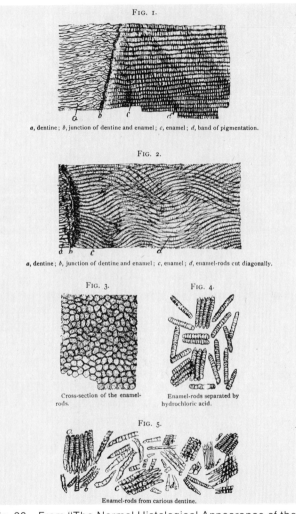

FIG. 1.

a, dentine; *b*, junction of dentine and enamel; *c*, enamel; *d*, band of pigmentation.

FIG. 2.

a, dentine; *b*, junction of dentine and enamel; *c*, enamel; *d*, enamel-rods cut diagonally.

FIG. 3.

FIG. 4.

Cross-section of the enamel-rods.

Enamel-rods separated by hydrochloric acid.

FIG. 5.

Enamel-rods from carious dentine.

Fig. 36   From "The Normal Histological Appearance of the Enamel," *Dental Cosmos* 33:1-14, 85-100, 347-358, 440-447, 526-543, 1891.

FIG. 6.

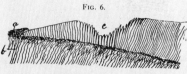

Diagram illustrating the beginning of caries on the labial surface of a central incisor. *a*, cementum overlapping the gingival margin of the enamel; *b*, dentine; *c*, beginning of caries, showing the enamel-rods separated by solution of cementing substance and partially broken away.

FIG. 7.

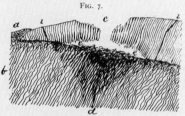

Diagram representing caries in the labial surface of a central incisor at a later stage than in Fig. 6. *a*, cementum; *b*, dentine; *c*, breach in the enamel; *d*, caries in the dentine, with the expansion of the tubules reaching toward the central part in the form of a cone; *e, e,* extension of the carious process between the dentine and enamel; *i, i,* lines upon which the margins of enamel should be formed in preparing for filling.

FIG. 8.

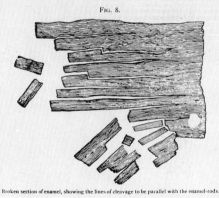

Broken section of enamel, showing the lines of cleavage to be parallel with the enamel-rods.

Fig. 37   Illustrations from "The Management of Enamel Margins," *Dental Cosmos,* 1891.

FIG. 9.

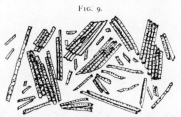

Parings from enamel made with a sharp chisel, holding its edge parallel with the enamel-rods.

FIG. 10.

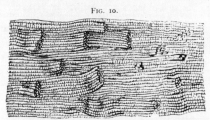

Split section of the enamel, showing its cleavage.

FIG. 11.

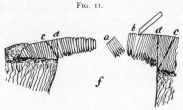

Diagram illustrating cleavage of the enamel and lines upon which the margin should be cut preparatory to filling. *a*, chip thrown off by the chisel; *b*, position of the chisel in splitting off overhanging margins; *c, c*, correct lines upon which to cut the margins preparatory to filling; *d, d*, incorrect lines for the preparation of the margins for filling; *f*, cavity in the dentine.

Fig. 38 Illustrations from part I of "The Management of Enamel Margins."

in Relation to Recurrence of Caries after Filling." The famous opening paragraphs of this important article are shown in Figure 40.

Black developed a scientifically based system of cavity preparation which proscribed new minimum cavity outline form extension limits - an expansion of the old limits - for the desired outline form of cavity preparations. The newly established extension limits required a cavity preparation outline form which included - and thus removed - all of the pits and central grooves and fissures in the enamel of the occlusal surfaces of the teeth. This new outline form also extended the interproximal margins of cavity preparations - and thus all of the margins of restorations - to a strategic location on each of the involved surfaces of the teeth where the enamel margins would be self-cleansed by the soft tissues of the mouth (Fig. 41).

Amalgam Research

The Society of Dental Surgeons in America in 1845 resolved to expel any of its members who used amalgam for a filling material. The most likely reason for this action by the Society was the poor quality of the many alloys which were then available on the market.

From 1883 to 1895, G. V. Black had been quietly and steadily conducting experiments on the use of amalgam as a filling material, and he had come to a different conclusion about the worth of amalgam. As a result of his studies with amalgam, Black believed that if amalgam was scientifically manufactured and scientifically utilized by dentists, amalgam was destined to serve well as a permanent filling material.

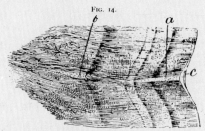

FIG. 14.

Section through the disto-buccal groove on the buccal surface of a lower first molar. *a,* Point of junction of the enamel-plates where the rods are spread apart and the space filled with granular material; *b,* A similar fault deeper in the enamel; *c,* A thickened portion of Nasmyth's membrane covering the groove.

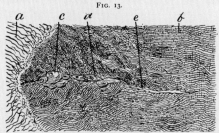

FIG. 13.

Section across the junction of the enamel-plates of an upper bicuspid cut on a line from the summit of the buccal cusp to the angle. *a,* Dentine; *b,* Enamel; *c,* Globular masses of calcific material in the line of junction of the enamel-plates; *d,* Long-shaped bodies; *e,* Hyaline material between the enamel-rods. The illustration shows only about half the thickness of the enamel. The surface half was regularly formed, and the apparent groove only a slight depression.

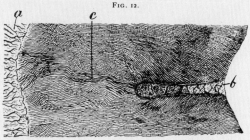

FIG. 12.

Section across the buccal groove of a lower first molar on a line between the cusps. *a,* Dentine; *b,* A fissure in the enamel closed with calcific material; *c,* Imperfect structure along the line of junction of the enamel-plates.

Schewe* has written: "His study of amalgam was exacting, requiring new instruments, which he himself made. In 1896, he gave us the first formula for a scientifically balanced amalgam, for he knew the secrets of expansion and contraction and he might have controlled its manufacture, commercialized his work, and enriched himself financially. But he did not. He (G. V. Black) was a professional man, a scientist and educator. 'He would not let die in him the man; he would not let perish the buds of art, poetry and science as they have died already in a thousand thousand men . . .' He would place his formula in the hands of the manufacturers. He called them together, and, for a small fee, gave them courses of lectures and demonstrated the making of a balanced alloy. His formula revolutionized dental practice. To illustrate: The Office of the Surgeon General stated that from December 7, 1941, to September 1, 1945, army dentists inserted 68,170,326 permanent restorations and most of them were amalgam."

Dean of Northwestern

The ability to teach other people was one of G. V. Black's many innate possessions, and it therefore followed quite naturally that he studied the problems of education. From 1870 he had taught at five dental schools, including Northwestern, where he began to teach in 1891. The dental schools at which he lectured

*Schewe, p. 20

Fig. 39   Illustrations from "Weak Lines of the Enamel," from part II of "The Management of Enamel Margins."

EXTENSION FOR PREVENTION, OR POSITION OF ENAMEL MARGINS CONSIDERED IN RELATION TO RECURRENCE OF CARIES AFTER FILLING.

When a cavity has occurred in the occluding surface of a molar, the dentist prepares for filling with the idea that the fissures in this part of the enamel have favored the occurrence of the cavity. For this reason the fissures and grooves adjoining the cavity, even though not decayed, are cut away to such a point as seems to give opportunity for a smooth, even finish of the margins of the filling. This is done as a prevention of future recurrence of decay, because such points have been observed to be more liable to caries than the smooth parts of the enamel. I think this has become a fixed principle with the large majority of operators ; and a failure to do this is regarded as careless operating. The sacrifice of the tooth-substance necessary is more than justifiable,—it is required for the safety of the operation and the tooth.

But why cut away such points? However the answer may be given, the principle is *extension for prevention*, or the removal of the enamel margin by cutting from a point of greater liability to a point of lesser liability to recurrence of caries. This principle is capable of a much wider range of usefulness than obtains at present, for, if my observation is correct, its use is confined almost exclusively to the grinding-surfaces by a large majority of operators. It seems that the thought has been, extension for a smooth finish, rather than the broader principle of extension for prevention.

It may be stated as an axiom that when reasonable extension of a cavity beyond the limits of present caries will appreciably diminish the dangers of recurrence, it should be done. A large proportion of decays occur in the proximate surfaces of the teeth ; and for many years it has been noted that recurrence of decay after filling is especially liable to occur in these surfaces. A reason for this has generally been sought in some fault in the management of the enamel margins. The enamel margins about a filling should always be regarded as a weak point, and should be guarded in every possible way against the dangers of recurrence of decay. One great difficulty has been that the same rule of extension for prevention has not been applied to the proximate surfaces as has obtained in the grinding-surfaces. In this case the obvious necessity of finding a point for a smooth finish has been lacking ; for on the proximate surfaces a smooth finish can be made at any point. Therefore, only the principle of removal of caries and cutting for anchorage has obtained.

Fig. 40   Black's statement of the epochal "Extension for Prevention," *Dental Cosmos* 33(2): 1891.

Fig. 41   Limits of ideal extension, as proposed by Black.

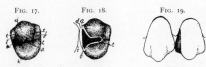

FIG. 17.   FIG. 18.   FIG. 19.

FIG. 17. Upper first bicuspid with cavity in the mesial surface. *a*, Buccal cusp ; *b*, Lingual cusp ; *c*, Distal groove ; *d*, Central groove ; *e, e*, Triangular grooves, mesial and distal ; *f, f*, Marginal ridges, mesial and distal ; *m*, Carious cavity.

FIG. 18. Same tooth as in Fig. 17, but with cavity prepared for filling. *a*, Mesio-buccal angle cut away to triangular groove ; *b*, Mesio-lingual angle cut away to a line that will be self-cleansing ; *c*, Shallow slot in the line of the central groove for anchorage ; *d*, Line of contour of filling ; *e*, Line of contour of the cuspid. The lines *d* and *e* show the form of proximate contact.

FIG. 19. The same teeth as in Fig. 18, after filling, in outline from the buccal surface, showing the form of contact and the interproximate space.

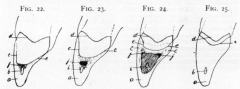

FIG. 22.   FIG. 23.   FIG. 24.   FIG. 25.

Figures 22, 23, 24, and 25 represent the proximate surfaces of an incisor with progressive recession of the gum septum. *a*, angle ; *b*, contact point ; *d*, gingival line, or line of attachment of the soft tissues to the neck of the tooth ; *e, e*, line of the free margin of the gum. In Fig. 22 this is almost complete ; reaching nearly to the point of contact, and covering a large portion of the proximate surface. The figures show progressive recession of the gum septum until in Fig. 25 the recession is extreme. *f*, in 22 and 23, shows the usual point of initial penetration of the enamel by caries ; and the shaded portions, areas of corrosion of the enamel in connection with the recession of the gum shown. Fig. 24, *b*, new point of contact on the filling, which later is shaded by dark lines ; *f, f*, points of recurring decay. The shading in dots shows the area exposed to corrosion by the recession of the gum septum shown by the line *e, e*. *c, c*, dotted line showing where the enamel margins should have been placed to prevent recurrence of caries.

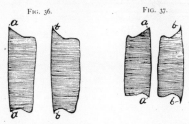

FIG. 36.   FIG. 37.

FIG. 36. Enlarged outline of filling, showing the margins as formed when the marginal edges of the enamel had been finished correctly and incorrectly. *a, a*, margins as formed when the marginal edge of the enamel is cut to a definite angle ; *b, b*, margins of the filling as formed when the angles of the marginal edge of the enamel have been slightly rounded with polishing powders.

FIG. 37. *a, a*, Form of the angles of the filling when the marginal edge of the enamel has been correctly finished ; *b, b*, form of the angles of the filling when the angles of the marginal edges of the enamel have been rounded by the use of emery in finishing. It will be noted that in each of these the angles *a, a*, are firm and definite, while the angles *b, b*, have thin feather edges which are unreliable.

were the Missouri Dental College, 1870-80; Chicago Dental Infirmary, 1883-85; Chicago College of Dental Surgery (later to become known as Northwestern University Dental School), 1885-90; Dental Department of the University of Iowa, 1890-91; and Northwestern University Dental School, 1891-1915.[*]

When G. V. Black began to teach at Northwestern University Dental School in 1891, he was Professor of Dental Pathology and Bacteriology; in 1893 he served as Chairman of the Section on Etiology, Pathology, and Bacteriology at the World's Columbian Dental Congress. He also delivered a "Report on Dental Nomenclature" at that Congress.[**]

In 1897 G. V. Black became Dean of Northwestern University Dental School. His official title then became "Dean and Professor of Operative Dentistry, Dental Pathology, and Bacteriology." In this capacity, he rendered dedicated service to dental education and the dental profession for seventeen years (Fig. 42).

"He had a particular faculty of allowing all minor details of family and profession to solve themselves. It often appeared that he took no interest in such matters. This was not the fact . . . He felt something of the same responsibility for the great professional family that he did for his own family."[***] (Fig. 43).

In 1897 too, he was elected President of the National School of Dental Technics, and in 1900 Black was elected President of the National Dental Association.

The First Fellowship Gold Medal was awarded by the Dental Society of the State of New York, in 1905, to G. V. Black.

[*]Black and Black, p. 344
[**]Dunning, p. 412
[***]Black and Black, p. 309

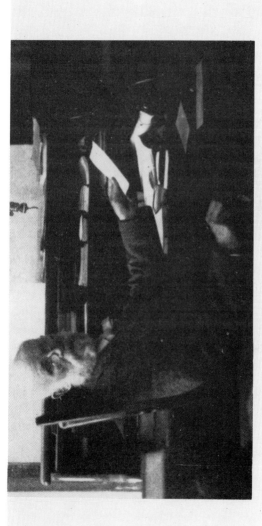

G. V. BLACK IN THE DEAN'S OFFICE AT NORTHWESTERN UNIVERSITY DENTAL SCHOOL.

Figure 42

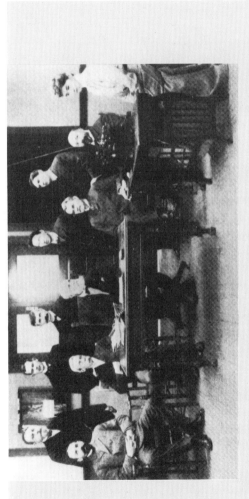

Dean G. V. Black presiding at a Faculty Meeting (about 1890). Left to right—(*seated*) Twing B. Wiggin, Edmund Noyes, G. V. Black, Thomas L. Gilmer, Wm. E. Harper, Emly Parr, secretary (*standing*) Benjamin Walberg, Benjamin Sellery, E. S. Willard, Frederick B. Noyes, Fred W. Gethro.

Figure 43

The American Dental Society of Europe invited Dr. Black to be a Special Guest at its Annual Meeting in 1906.

"In 1908, in addition to his lectures at the dental school and sixteen papers, with the best paper, printing, and illustrating available, Black's monumental two-volume work, Operative Dentistry, was published. This work was the magnificent scientific and artistic culmination of his long labors "[*] (Figs. 44-52).

G. V. Black began Volume 2, "Technical Procedures in Filling Teeth," with a description of his system of cavity nomenclature in order that better teacher-student communication would result.

The next chapter of this volume was titled "Cutting Instruments." Black used the carpentry nomenclature system (class name, instrument formula) to name operative dental hand instruments, e.g., bibeveled hatch-(et, 3-1-28); this system is still in use today. The measurements following the instrument class names (i.e., chisel, hatchet, hoe, etc.), called the instrument formula; were necessary for instant identification of instruments. The formula described the blade with the following numbers: (1) width - in tenths of millimeters, (2) length - in millimeters, (3) angle of the blade - in degrees. The correct design for contra-angled hand instruments was included in the illustrations of instruments in this chapter (Fig. 48).

In addition to discussing the correct use of dental hand instruments and the proper use of the rubber dam, Black discussed the "Histological Structure of the Teeth in Relation to Cavity Preparation." The emphasis in this chapter is on the location of the recessional

[*]Ibid., pp. 303-306

A WORK

ON

OPERATIVE DENTISTRY

IN TWO VOLUMES.

VOLUME ONE,

THE PATHOLOGY OF THE HARD TISSUES OF THE TEETH.

GLOSSARY AND INDEX.

187 ILLUSTRATIONS.

BY

G. V. BLACK, M.D., D.D.S., Sc.D., LL.D.

DEAN AND PROFESSOR OF OPERATIVE DENTISTRY, DENTAL PATHOLOGY AND BACTERIOLOGY
NORTHWESTERN UNIVERSITY DENTAL SCHOOL.

1908.

MEDICO-DENTAL PUBLISHING COMPANY,
CHICAGO

lines of the pulpal horns and the direction of the enamel rods. True, then, as now, it is important for the dentist to be aware of the location of the recessional lines of the pulpal horns in order to prevent inadvertent exposure of the pulp during cavity preparation. It is also necessary to be aware of the direction of the enamel rods so that the enamel margins of cavity preparations can be prepared correctly.

After discussing the injuries to the teeth by caries (Figs. 49, 50) Black listed the seven certain fundamental principles of cavity preparation.

1. Obtain the required outline form.
2. Obtain the required retention form.
3. Obtain the required resistance form.
4. Obtain the required convenience form.
5. Remove any remaining carious dentin.
6. Finish the enamel wall.
7. Make the toilet of the cavity.

Steps two and three were combined in later editions of this book.

Fig. 44 Title page of the first volume of the first edition. With very few exceptions, the illustrations were prepared by G. V. Black. Dr. Arthur D. Black revised the work six times, under the title "G. V. Black's Work on Operative Dentistry with Which His Special Dental Pathology Is Combined" and Dr. Robert E. Blackwell revised it for the seventh time in 1955, under the title "G. V. Black's Operative Dentistry." The last edition remained in print until the advent of ultra high-speed dental handpieces which require different operative techniques.

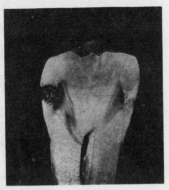

Fɪɢ. 117.

Fɪɢ. 117. This excellent photograph of a split bicuspid with mesial and distal decays is remarkably similar to the last, but in many ways a more perfect picture than Figure 114. In the decay on the left, the enamel rods are broken down and are lying in the cavity in the enamel in a tangled mass. In the decay on the right, the enamel rods are still in perfect position and no microörganisms have been admitted to the dentin. The dark portion of the dentin accurately exhibits actual decay of the dentin in both decays. The hyaline areas are both very well shown. The forked projection of the flamelike tongue on the left, formed by the border of cloud, is one of the singularly interesting features.

Fig. 45   Carious decay, as illustrated by Black. "In the decay on the left, the enamel rods are broken down and are lying in the cavity in the enamel in a tangled mass. In the decay on the right, the enamel rods are still in perfect position and no microorganisms have been admitted to the dentin. The dark portion of the dentin accurately exhibits actual decay of the dentin . . ." From vol., 2, "A Work on Operative Dentistry."

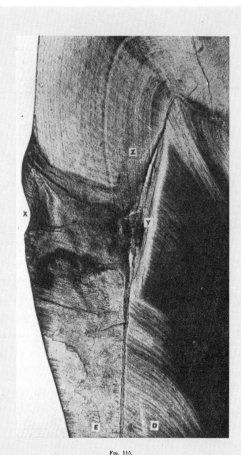

Fig. 115.

Fig. 115. Photomicrograph showing the carious area seen on the left of the small photograph, Figure 114. D. Dentin. E. Enamel. X. Area of decay. Y. Line of actual solution of the calcium salts of the dentin. Z. Backward decay of the enamel, which shows very white by reflected light, but is dark by transmitted light. In the drying of the specimen, the decayed dentin has shrunken and pulled a little away from the enamel. A slight break of the enamel rods has occurred at X, and a little confusion of the decayed rods has occurred near the letter Y. No enamel rods have fallen out, however, and microörganisms have not been admitted to the dentin.

Fig. 46 Another micrographic view of caries attack, from the same source.

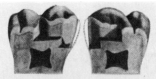

Fig. 6.

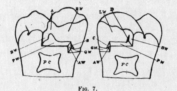

Fig. 7.

Fig. 6. An upper first molar with a prepared mesio-occlusal cavity, split mesio-distally, displaying the cavity form. The buccal half is on the left and the lingual half on the right side. The mesial surfaces of the two halves are next each other. The dotted lines rounding from these show the form of the mesial surface of the filling if it were placed.

Fig. 7. An outline view of the cavity shown in Figure 6 for a further study of the internal parts. D w. Distal wall. P w. Pulpal wall. G w. Gingival wall. A w. Axial wall. B w. Buccal wall. L w. Lingual wall. P c. Pulp chamber. A. Acute angle formed by cutting out the buccal groove. D. Convenience point cut in the disto-linguo-pulpal angle. B. Convenience point cut in the bucco-axio-gingival angle. C. Convenience point cut in the linguo-axio-gingival angle.

Fig. 47 Illustrations from "The Technical Procedures in Filling Teeth," volume 2 of "A Work on Operative Dentistry." At a banquet in 1910, Thomas Gilmer reported that he had observed "mechanical drawings on the walls" of Black's laboratory during his first visit to the Black office in Jacksonville. Black regularly used vertical and horizontal section and surface view drawings of cavity preparations and restorations. Orthographic projection of this sort is of great value for describing interior detail of objects such as cavity preparations.

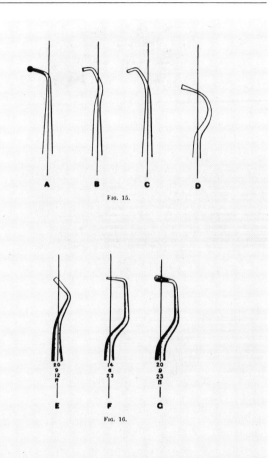

Fig. 15.

Fig. 16.

Fig. 15. Instruments wrongly contra-angled. Their points are so far from the line of the central axis of the shaft, as shown by the line, that they incline to twist, or turn, in the fingers when the effort is made to cut with them. They are out of balance.

Fig. 16. Instruments correctly contra-angled. Their points are brought close enough to the line of the central axis so that they will not be inclined to twist, or turn, in the fingers when the effort is made to cut with them. They are well balanced.

Fig. 48   Additional illustrations from "A Work on Operative Dentistry."

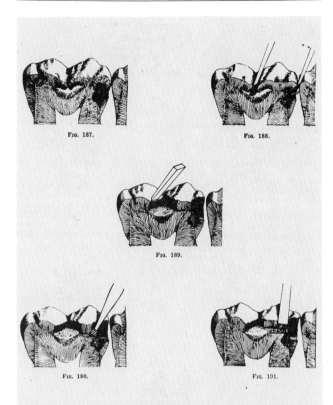

FIGS. 187-196. A series of ten pen pictures illustrating methods of excavating deep mesio-occlusal cavities and avoiding pulp exposure. The tooth is cut mesio-distally and only the buccal half is used. The dento-enamel-junction is made diagrammatically prominent. The cut is, of course, not in the line of any of the horns of the pulp, but the recessional line of the mesial crest of the margin of the pulp is darkened for a space, representing the probable length of the mesio-buccal horn of the pulp.

FIG. 187. The buccal half of a lower molar split mesio-distally, displaying a cavity in the occlusal surface and an independent cavity in the mesial surface. In the case of a young person with the large pulp chamber at that age, these cavities should be regarded as seriously endangering the pulp.

FIG. 188. The chisel in position for beginning chipping away the undermined enamel over each of the decayed areas. The first chip is represented as broken away in each.

FIG. 189. Represents the progress in chipping away the undermined enamel with the chisel in position for removing the distal portion by the pulling motion.

FIG. 190. The inverted cone bur 10 in position for cutting a slot through the sound portion of enamel between the two cavities.

FIG. 191. The chisel or enamel hatchet removing the enamel undermined by the bur, widening the slot.

Fig. 49   Illustrations from "Technical Procedures in Filling Teeth," 1908.

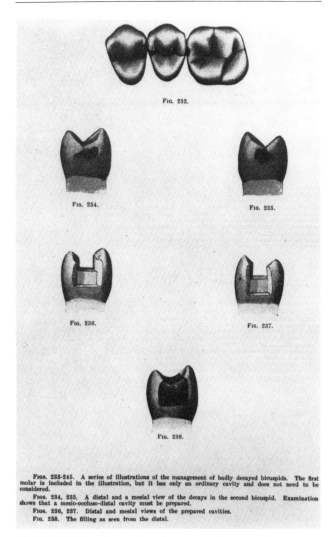

Fig. 233.

Fig. 234.

Fig. 235.

Fig. 236.

Fig. 237.

Fig. 238.

Figs. 233-245. A series of illustrations of the management of badly decayed bicuspids. The first molar is included in the illustration, but it has only an ordinary cavity and does not need to be considered.

Figs. 234, 235. A distal and a mesial view of the decays in the second bicuspid. Examination shows that a mesio-occluso-distal cavity must be prepared.

Figs. 236, 237. Distal and mesial views of the prepared cavities.

Fig. 238. The filling as seen from the distal.

Fig. 50 Outline form of cavity preparations and a restoration, (from "A Work on Operative Dentistry").

In the "Technical Procedures," Black described the "Excavation of Cavities by Classes." The classes are:

Class 1. Cavities beginning in the structural defects in the teeth, pits, fissures.

Class 2. Cavities in the proximal surfaces of the premolars and molars.

Class 3. Cavities in the proximal surfaces of the incisors which do not involve the removal and restoration of the incisal angle.

Class 4. Cavities in the proximal surfaces of the incisors which do require the removal and restoration of the incisal angle.

Class 5. Cavities in the gingival third - not pit cavities of the labial, buccal, or lingual surfaces of the teeth.

Other chapter titles of this book were "Physical Properties of Filling Materials and Correlation of Forces Concerned," "Filling with Gold," "Filling Cavities with Gold by Classes," and "Amalgam" (includes a historical review and principles governing its correct use). There is a chapter on "Porcelain and Gold Inlays" and also a chapter on "The Cements." Technical Procedures in Filling Teeth comes to an end with a review of the techniques for the removal of the dental pulp and the filling of root canals (Figs. 51-53).

In 1909 he prepared twenty-six papers. Some of the titles were:

Supernumerary Teeth. Indiana State Den. Soc. Dental Summary, Vol. 29, 1909, p. 1, 83. 90 Illus.

Gold Fillings. Discussion. Penn. State Den. Soc. Dental Cosmos, Vol. 51, 1909, p. 1307.

Mastication and Insalivation of Food. Den. Soc. State N.Y. Dental Cosmos, Vol. 51, 1909, p. 1187.

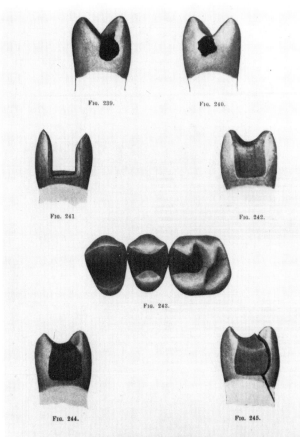

Figs. 239, 240. Distal and mesial views of the first bicuspid, showing the decays. Examination reveals extensive exposure of the pulp, which must be removed.

Fig. 241. The prepared cavity. Notice that the enamel has been cut away just over the points of the cusps.

Fig. 242. The cavity filled. Notice that the filling material protects the entire occlusal surface so that the danger of the cusps being split off by the wedging of food between them is removed.

Fig. 243. The finished case as seen from the occlusal view.

Fig. 244. A view of the first bicuspid, as often filled, in mesio-occlusal-distal cavities after removal of the pulp, which gives the appearance of a much better tooth.

Fig. 245. This exhibits the usual result of a filling placed as shown in Figure 244, which, sooner or later, is pretty sure to occur from the wedging of food between the cusps.

Fig. 51   More outline forms, same source.

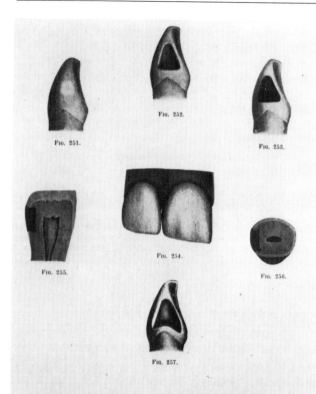

FIGS. 251-257. A series illustrating the minimum and maximum cavity extension in incisor proximal cavities.

FIG. 251. The distal surface of a central incisor with a decay in which the enamel rods have just begun to fall away. There is practically no burrowing of decay in the dentin, though some softening has occurred. No matter what the extension demanded to prevent recurrence of decay, no part of this cavity needs to be cut deeper than may be required for safe anchorage.

FIG. 252. The cavity preparation, exhibiting a minimum extension, and the outline form that should generally be used.

FIG. 253. The finished filling.

FIG. 254. The finished filling as seen from the labial.

FIG. 255. Mesio-distal section of the tooth and the filling, showing the depth of cutting and the incisal anchorage.

FIG. 256. A cross section of the tooth and the filling close to the gingival wall, showing the retention in the gingival portion.

FIG. 257. A cavity preparation showing extreme extension. Practically the extension for prevention in incisor cavities should always be kept between this and that shown in Figure 252. Its amount should depend upon the conditions demanding extension in each particular case. A filling made after the cavity preparation in Figure 257 would be seen from the labial very little more than that in Figure 254.

Fig. 52 Outline forms and restorations for anterior teeth, same source.

Our Little Patients. Discussion. Chicago-Odontographic Soc. Dental Review, Vol. 23, 1909, p. 92.

First Permanent Molar. Discussion. Chicago-Odontographic Soc. Dental Review, Vol. 23, 1909, p. 268, 278.

Dental Science and Literature. Discussion. Ill. S. Den. Soc. Transactions, 1909, p. 39. Dental Review, Vol. 23, 1909, p. 679.

The Possibilities of Closer Cooperation between the Dental and Medical Professions. Discussion. Ill. S. Den. Soc. Transactions, 1909, p. 112. Dental Review, Vol. 23, 1909, p. 856.

Investigation of Mottled Enamel. Chicago-Odontographic Soc. September, 1909. Not published.

A Plea for Greater Earnestness in the Study of Caries of the Enamel in its Relation to the Practice of Dentistry. Academy of Stomatology, Philadephia. Nov., 1909. Not published.

In 1910, the Chicago Odontographic Society held a testimonial banquet in honor of Dr. Black.

Also in 1910, The *Fédération Dentaire Internationale* awarded its first W. D. Miller Award of $10,000 ($8,000 of which was contributed by European sources and $2,000 by Americans) together with a gold medal to Dr. G.V. Black for his outstanding contributions to dentistry. The award was presented at the London meeting on August 1, 1911, and:

It was rapid recognition in the field of science, an expression of the broad-minded spirit of its European founders, and a reward to G. V. Black for fifty-three years of hard work.*

Professor Hubert Anson Newton described the happiness and satisfaction which is experienced in doing creative work. He said:

*Black and Black, p. 311

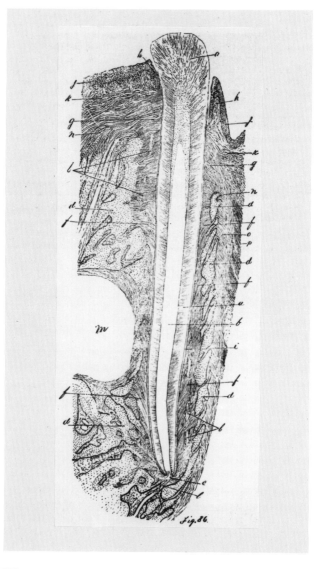

Fig. 86.

Fig. 36, 2 in. obj. Lengthwise section of small incisor tooth of kitten with its membrane and alveolus. The portion included in the illustration is one-fourth in. long. *a, a,* Crown of tooth and dentine. *b,* Pulp chamber and root canal. *c,* Cementum. *d, d, d, d,* Alveolar walls. *e,* Apical space and apical foramen. *f, f, f, f,* Body of peridental membrane, showing particularly the arrangement of its principal fibers, their direction, etc. *g, g,* The cervical portion of the peridental membrane, showing the relation of its fibers to the gingivus *h,* the tangled mass of fibers forming the gums *k,* and the periosteum *n, n,* of the outer surface of alveolar wall. *h, h,* Gingivus. *j, j,* Epithelium. *k, k,* Coarse fibrous tissue of the gums. *l, l, l,* Bloodvessels traversing the peridental membrane. A section showing the smallest number of these was selected, for the reason that the fibrous arrangement is less distorted. *m,* Saculus of permanent tooth. The fibers of the peridental membrane become continuous with those of the periosteum at *n, n. o,* Periosteum. *p,* Attachment of labial muscles. The intention of the illustration is to give a full view of the arrangement of the fibers of the peridental membrane, and the relations of the tooth, membrane, and alveolar wall.

Fig. 53 (left and top) This illustration, originally published in Black's second book, was included as Fig. 25 in his last book, "A Work On Special Dental Pathology" (Medico-Dental Publishing Co., Chicago and Claudius Ash, Son & Co., London, 1915).

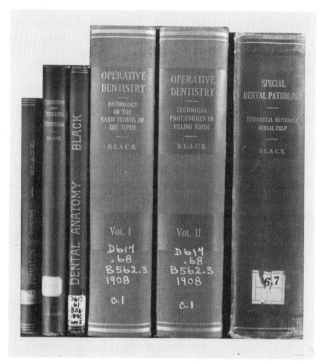

Fig. 54   Black's works.

"To discover some new truth in nature, . . . gives one of the purest pleasures in human experience. It gives joy to tell others of the treasures found."[*]

On April 12, 1915, after five years of preparation, G. V. Black published Special Dental Pathology, which was to be his last book (Fig. 54). From 1864 to 1915 he had produced more than 1,300 papers and addresses on

[*]Ruckeyser, p. 291

scientific and professional subjects . . . He became the foremost leader in dental education, and (as Dean of Northwestern) he helped build one of the leading dental schools in the world.*

Return to Walnut Grove

On the old farm, which he had named Walnut Grove Farm—after his father had died in 1884, and he had purchased his brothers' and other heirs' interests in this land—where he had spent his boyhood and also many restful vacations of the latter years of his life, G. V. Black died on August 31, 1915.

"From all parts of the world came messages of tribute to his transcendent ability, his superlative contributions and unselfish devotion."**

A bust of G. V. Black made by Professor Salvadore De Simons of Naples, Italy, was presented to Dr. Arthur D. Black by Gr. Uff. Dott. Vincenzo Guerini of Naples. A statue of G. V. Black, erected by the American Dental Association in G. V. Black's favorite part of Lincoln Park in Chicago, Illinois, was unveiled on August 7, 1918; and at Winchester, Illinois, on October 16, 1930, there was placed a tablet dedicated to Greene Vardiman Black with the inscription:

GREENE VARDIMAN BLACK
1836-1915
Father of Modern Dentistry
Born In Scott County, Illinois
His First Office (1857)
Was on Lot 64, This Square

*Schewe, p. 20
**Ibid., p. 20

In 1965, G. V. Black's name was carved into the frieze of the new addition to the Centennial Building of the State of Illinois in Springfield.

Chapter 5

Service

G. V. Black's most famous book, A Work on Operative Dentistry, went through nine editions in English, all of which were sold out. It was translated into other languages, and it remained in print in the English language and rendered admirable service to the dental profession for more than fifty years.

'Caritas'

The beneficial effects and enduring service of G. V. Black's works (Figs. 55-59) should perhaps be attributed more to the spirit in which he approached his work than to any other single factor. One of his friends once said that he could not see the need for all of G. V. Black's burning of the midnight oil. Somewhat later, another friend commented that G. V. Black had been financially independent for a long time and that his circumstances did not require his extensive activity on behalf of the dental profession. We are fortunate that he chose to be so busy.

Caritas, the Latin word for charity, seems to describe most closely his love, primarily for both the essence of his work in dentistry itself, and for dentistry's beneficent service to the public. For G. V. Black, as the night-the day, did the rewards - spiritual, material and professional - soon follow this genuine spirit of *caritas.*

THE

FORMATION OF POISONS

BY

MICRO-ORGANISMS.

A BIOLOGICAL STUDY OF THE GERM THEORY OF DISEASE.

BY

G. V. BLACK, M.D., D.D.S.

PHILADELPHIA:
P. BLAKISTON, SON & CO.,
No. 1012 WALNUT STREET.
1884.

Figure 55

A STUDY

OF THE

HISTOLOGICAL CHARACTERS

OF THE

Periosteum and Peridental

MEMBRANE.

BY

G. V. BLACK, M.D., D.D.S.

PROFESSOR OF PATHOLOGY IN THE CHICAGO COLLEGE OF DENTAL SURGERY.

WITH 67 ORIGINAL ILLUSTRATIONS.

CHICAGO:
W. T. KEENER,
96 WASHINGTON STREET.
1887.

Figure 56

Descriptive Anatomy

OF THE

Human Teeth.

BY

G. V. BLACK, M.D., D.D.S.

PUBLISHED BY
THE WILMINGTON DENTAL MANUFACTURING CO.
1413 FILBERT STREET,
PHILADELPHIA, PA.
Copyrighted, 1890, by The Wilmington Dental M'f'g Co., Phila.

Figure 57

A WORK

ON

OPERATIVE DENTISTRY

IN TWO VOLUMES.

VOLUME TWO,

THE TECHNICAL PROCEDURES IN FILLING TEETH.

INDEX.

---

437 ILLUSTRATIONS.

BY

G. V. BLACK, M.D., D.D.S., Sc.D., LL.D.

DEAN AND PROFESSOR OF OPERATIVE DENTISTRY, DENTAL PATHOLOGY AND BACTERIOLOGY
NORTHWESTERN UNIVERSITY DENTAL SCHOOL.

1908.

MEDICO-DENTAL PUBLISHING COMPANY.

CHICAGO.

Figure 58

A WORK

ON

SPECIAL DENTAL PATHOLOGY

DEVOTED TO THE

DISEASES AND TREATMENT

OF THE

INVESTING TISSUES OF THE TEETH AND THE DENTAL PULP

INCLUDING THE SEQUELÆ OF THE DEATH OF THE PULP;
ALSO, SYSTEMIC EFFECTS OF MOUTH INFECTIONS,
ORAL PROPHYLAXIS AND MOUTH HYGIENE

518 ILLUSTRATIONS

BY

G. V. BLACK, M.D., D.D.S., SC.D., LL.D.

DEAN AND PROFESSOR OF OPERATIVE DENTISTRY, DENTAL PATHOLOGY AND BACTERIOLOGY
NORTHWESTERN UNIVERSITY DENTAL SCHOOL

1915

MEDICO-DENTAL PUBLISHING COMPANY
CHICAGO

CLAUDIUS ASH, SONS & COMPANY
LONDON

Figure 59

Advances and New Perspectives in Operative Dentistry

Just as G. V. Black had predicted, the future brought about many changes in the practice of dentistry and in operative dentistry in particular. One of the early chapters of "The Technical Procedures in Filling Teeth" was "Positions at the Chair." Maximum comfort of both patient and dentist was the objective described. In attempting to reach this goal of maximum comfort during operative procedures, Black had devised a cocaine-pressure method for anesthetizing individual teeth after cavity preparation had begun. Later, local anesthetics, of which procaine was the first, were introduced to dental practice. With its introduction, it was often possible to anesthetize several teeth with a single injection before cavity preparation was begun. It was possible now to carry out cavity preparation painlessly from the beginning.

Introduction, in the mid-1950's, of time and motion principles to dental office design and practice was the next major step toward the goal Black suggested. Among the innovations in dental practice arising from these studies were efficient office traffic patterns resulting from improved office design, and more conveniently located dental units. Better quality of dental treatment for patients in less time with less stress resulted from the use of washed field procedures in systematized operating routines. Both patient and operating team could be more relaxed and free of tension with the introduction of contour dental chairs, standardized instrument operating trays, and fully adjustable dentist and dental assistant operating stools. As the patient now was in a relaxed, reclined position, the operating team worked in a more organized manner from the more comfortable seated position. This team technique of dental practice, with trained dental auxiliary assistance constantly at chairside, has become known as "four-handed dentistry." Such ergonomic advances resulted in reduced fatigue as well as increased productivity for the dentist; for dental patients, they resulted in less stressful dental appointments, with improved dental health and physical well-being attainable in a shorter time than ever before.

It is in the subject of cavity preparation, however, where the greatest changes in thinking in operative dentistry have occurred since the time of G. V. Black. In general, dentists continue to believe that the basic principles of cavity preparation which were established by G. V. Black remain valid today, but that they need to be modified to bring them into harmony with the advances and new perspectives which have been gained in operative dentistry theory and technique.*

Chief among the reasons for the need to modify these principles are the advances and improvements which have been made in (1) cutting instruments - the advent of the ultra high-speed hand pieces and the improvements which have been made in dental burs, (2) dental filling and impression materials, and (3) increased public awareness of the causes of dental caries and the important role of the individual patient in practicing self-control of tooth decay preventive measures.

In G. V. Black's principle of extension for prevention, perhaps more than in any aspect of his work, have the advances in these three areas brought the dental profession to a new perspective in operative dentistry - specifically in the areas of outline form extension and

*Welk and Laswell

in the internal design of cavity preparations. The introduction of the ultra high-speed hand piece to the dental profession in the late 1950's permitted a much more efficient and less heat-generating preparation of cavities. With ultra high-speed cutting techniques, it was no longer necessary for the dentist to depend on the previously indispensable inverted cone bur for undermining the enamel at the dento-enamel junction before cleaving the enamel rods with a hand instrument, as illustrated in Black's "Technical Procedures" (Fig. 49). Before the introduction of ultra high-speed operating techniques, for over fifty years this technique of undermining and cleaving the enamel was the most rapid method of removing tooth structure. With ultra high-speed operating methods that required the operator to use the dental handpiece with a brushlike, light-pressured painting motion, cavity preparation could be accomplished with much greater efficiency and much less generation of heat by using slender, round-tipped, plain, tapered fissure burs. Cavity preparations whose internal line angles are more rounded rather than sharp now could be prepared. More rounded line angles, where indicated in cavity preparation, reduce the likelihood that undesirable stresses will be introduced into the restoration.

In 1891 in "The Management of Enamel Margins,"[*] Black identified the enamel margins as the weakest part of dental restorations. This is still true today. In "The Technical Procedures in Filling Teeth," which is Volume 2 of A Work on Operative Dentistry (1908), Black defined the "flow" of amalgam restorations as ". . . its disposition to move continuously under a given

[*] G. V. Black

fixed pressure." He also noted that any amalgam that will flow under a pressure of fifty pounds is unfit for filling teeth on that account. Flow of amalgam restorations over enamel margins can result in failure of the restorations due to fracture of the excess amalgam followed by leakage of mouth fluids at the enamel margins of the restorations. Micro-leakage of fluids at the enamel margins of dental restorations remains a serious problem and a challenge to clinicians and researchers in operative dentistry today.

Improved impression materials and controlled casting techniques have resulted in cast gold inlay restorations which possess precision adaptations at the enamel margins. The use of an unfilled resin to bond composite resin to enamel has resulted in stronger, highly aesthetic composite resin restorations for anterior teeth, with lower micro-leakage at the enamel margins than any other material which was used before the 1970's. The dental restorative material which produces the best adaptation to the enamel margins is cohesive gold foil. Two of the disadvantages of the use of this material are that it is difficult and time consuming to manipulate. This had tended to discourage its use as a filling material. In the 1970's, however, a manufactured product which consisted of mat gold wrapped in a cohesive gold foil covering was introduced as a direct filling gold restorative material. The use of cohesive gold foil has been greatly encouraged because, in the form of direct filling gold, this material is much easier and less time consuming to use.

Together with these developments in the late 1960's came the increased patient awareness and practice of self-control of dental caries and other dental and oral diseases. This advance was the result of emphasis on preventive home care, a major effort at patient education by the dental profession. Patient education was undoubtedly aided by television advertising of dentifrices and other dental home care devices.

These advances in operative dentistry have brought the dental profession to a new perspective in thinking about cavity preparation. With it has come a need to modify G. V. Black's principle of extension for prevention of the recurrence of the decay. Specifically, these advances have established a narrower range of limits - approximately one-quarter rather than one-third or more of the inter-cuspal distance - for the satisfactory location of the buccal and lingual enamel margins of cavity preparations on the occlusal surfaces and not more than explorer tip clearance from the adjacent tooth for the optimum location of the buccal, lingual, and gingival interproximal enamel margins of anterior as well as posterior teeth. These are the generally accepted maximum extension limits for ideal cavity preparation on normally aligned teeth with early carious lesions for a patient with good oral hygiene and conscientious home care.

Further modifications in the extension limits for cavity preparations may occur again in the future, but the objective still will be the same: After all of the dental caries have been removed, the outline form of the cavity preparation should be extended only so far as is necessary for the dentist to do everything possible to protect the tooth from recurrence of decay at the enamel margins and at the same time to produce a cavity preparation which will provide maximum conservation and strength of natural tooth structure as well as maximum strength and retention of the restoration, with minimum necessary extension (See Fig. 41).

Maximum prevention with minimum extension appears to be the trend in outline form extension for the cavity preparations which will be used in operative dentistry in the future.

In the introduction to the 1936 revision of A Work on Operative Dentistry, which was titled, G. V. Black's Work on Operative Dentistry, with which his Special Dental Pathology Is Combined, the editor, Dr. Arthur D. Black-G. V. Black's son-described the mission of his father's famous book:

"Operative Dentistry, in the author's conception, consists of all procedures, including preventive measures, by which the teeth may be conserved, and thus maintain the natural masticating mechanism in such a state that the general health will not be endangered."

Dr. Robert E. Blackwell, editor of the ninth edition of this book, which was now titled "G. V. Black's Operative Dentistry," in 1955, added:*

"The basic idea expressed in Volume I and continued in Volume II is that the natural dentures of nearly everyone can be conserved throughout the childhood period and, well into adult life, or until those degenerative processes set in over which we have little or no control."

These statements also perfectly and beautifully describe the purposeful mission of G. V. Black's life and work in dentistry which was recorded in A Work on Operative Dentistry (Fig. 58), his most famous book.

This book represented a giant step toward a lasting scientific solution to the American dental problem and even more universally, to the dental problem of all mankind.

*Blackwell, R.E.

One friend of G. V. Black recalled this happy memory: "I once had the rare pleasure of going with Dr. Black on one of his tramps across the fields and over the streams . . . everything seemed to grow and take on color when he spoke of it. He was an expert florist . . . There was such a simple relationship between him and nature. He was in harmony with the deep wood and the clear sky above him . . . he talked of the unending life behind the visible face of things, and what it would be like to live there, to get at the heart of all these mysteries; to see how truth is tied to truth . . . and to see how events grow out of each other and into each other."*

A hunting and fishing friend who was a jeweler in Jacksonville, Illinois, Mr. C. H. Russell, said of G. V. Black:

"I continually marveled at the wonderful knowledge he possessed, not only of all mechanical problems, but especially at his remarkable dexterity in the actual performance of any process necessary to the carrying out of his far reaching mechanical ideas. He was one who could not only 'make the machine but could also make the machine that made it.'"**

Dr. Edward F. Schewe makes this concluding remark about Black's long career—with these impressive words:

"It was universally recognized that, among the men who have stamped the impress of their greatness upon the profession of dentistry, the figure of the Immortal G. V. towers upward like a cathedral dome."***

There he is: G. V. Black the man (Fig. 60). He was a

*Obituary
**Black and Black, pp. 371-372
***Schewe, p. 20

man who, throughout his life, related himself to *nature*: first, through the art of direct experience and observation and later by self-continuing education through the study of deductively formulated *science*; secondly, he was a man who related himself to other people through service to his *community*; and thirdly, he was a man with an overarching *purpose* in his life. His purpose was to raise dentistry from its status of an obscure trade, in which he found it, to the level of a profession; and finally, through his published works, he rendered a continuing *service* by helping to greatly increase, in many ways, the public well-being and the stature of the dental profession for the benefit of the peoples of the world.

Science, community, purpose, and service! Dr. G. V. Black personified the spirit of these four themes, which have been "themes dominant" in American life and religious and philosophical thought at their best.

These are the things which he had accomplished, and yet, he still affects us today, in many ways. William B. Dunning prefaced his 1915 memoir, "Greene Vardiman Black," with this poem of Kipling:

Let us now praise famous men—
Men of little showing!
For their work continueth
And their work continueth,
Broad and deep continueth—
Great, beyond their knowing.

But perhaps the most recent way in which he affects us is in continuing education and, perhaps, it is the best way to remember him. In G. V. Black's own words:

> "The Professional Man has
> No right to be other than a
> Continuous student."

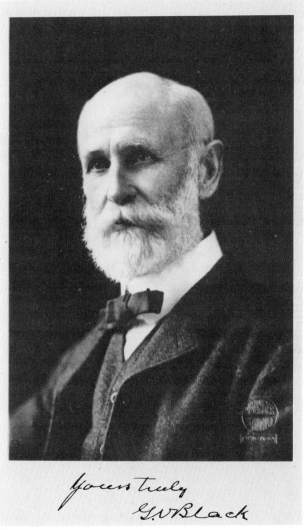

Figure 60

References

Anon. 1910. Honor to Dr. G. V. Black. *Northwestern Dent. J.* 7 (4): 111-42.

Black, A.D. (ed.) 1936. *G. V. Black's work on operative dentistry with which his special dental pathology is combined.* Chicago: Medico-Dental Publ.

Black, C. E. and Black, B. M. 1940. *From pioneer to scientist.* St. Paul: Bruce.

Black, Mrs. C. E. II. 1977. Personal communication.

Black, G. V. 1891. The management of enamel margins. *Dent. Cosmos.* 33: 1-14, 85-100, 347-58, 440-47, 526-43.

Blackwell, R.E. (ed.) 1955. *G. V. Black's operative dentistry.* South Milwaukee: Medico-Dental Publ.

Dubos, R. 1960. *Pasteur and modern science.* Garden City: Anchor Books, Doubleday.

Dunning, W. B. 1915. Greene Vardiman Black. *J. Allied Dent. Soc.* 10 (4): 409-17.

Fosdick, R., and Turner, F. 1929. In *Adventurous America,* ed. E. Mims. New York: Charles Scribner's Sons.

Northrop, F.S.C. (a) 1952. *The taming of the nations.* New York: MacMillan.

Northrop, F.S.C. (b) 1947. *The logic of the sciences and the humanities.* New York: MacMillan.

Obituary. 1915. Dr. Greene Vardiman Black. *Northwestern Dent. J.* 11 (8): 2-11.

Rukeyser, M. 1964. *Willard Gibbs.* New York: E.P. Dutton.

Schewe, E. F. 1951. *Aspects of professional life and other sketches.* Los Angeles: Institute Press.

Smith, J. E. ed. (a) 1970. *Signs, selves and interpretation. Contemporary American philosophy, Second Series.* George Allen and Unwin.

Smith, J. E. (b) 1970. *Themes in American philosophy.* New York: Harper & Row.

Thorpe, B. L. 1909. In *history of dental surgery.* Vol. 3 Ed. C.R.E. Koch. Chicago: National Art. Publ.

Welk, D.A. and Laswell, H.R. 1976. Rationale for designing cavity preparations in light of current knowledge and technology. *Dent. Clin. N. Amer.* 20: 231-39.